Life with Bipolar Type Two
a guide to stability

By

Eleanor Worsley

Eleanor Worsley

Disclaimer: The contents of this book are in no way meant to perform as a substitute or replacement for professional medical advice and treatment.

Copyright © 2019 Eleanor Worsley

Artwork Copyright © 2019 Irfon Rickard

All rights reserved.

ISBN: 9781689557375

CONTENTS

Contents
Introductions 1

Chapter One: 4

Bipolar in General 4

    What is Bipolar Disorder? 5

    What is Bipolar Type Two (BPII)? 7

    What Causes Bipolar Disorder? 9

    History of Bipolar: 12

    Diagnosis: 15

    Misdiagnosis: 16

    Children Whose Parents Have Bipolar Disorder: ...18

    Medical Conditions that Mimic BP Symptomology 19

Chapter Two: 21

Symptoms 21

    Depression 22

    Hypomania 28

    Anxiety 41

    Self-harm 50

    Suicide 55

    Sex & Hypersexuality 58

    Catastrophising 60

Chapter Three: 63

Treatment 63

    Without Treatment 64

- Psychiatrists 64
- Psychopharmacology (psychiatric medication) 71
- Psychology & Psychotherapy 94
- Complementary and Alternative Medicine...................... 101
- Advanced Directives.. 112

Chapter Four: 114

Management and Lifestyle 114

- Sleep... 115
- Stress... 118
- Exercise 123
- Diet.. 129
- Support Networks 132
- Telling People You Have Bipolar 137
- Friends with Mental Health Disorders 142
- Mindfulness.. 146
- Writing to Keep Us on Track 151
- Creativity.. 153
- Wasting Time with a Purpose 157

Chapter Five: 158

My Musings 158

- Wellness Language.. 159
- Bipolar Man's Best Friend: pets and mental illness 165
- My Bipolar Idols 167
- Bipolar: friend or foe? 169
- A Marathon of Sprints and Stops...................................... 171

A Reason, Not an Excuse 173

Stability is the Goal..174

If you're reading this book because it's a loved one who has BPII..180

Thank you 183

Thank You and Goodbye 183

Bibliography..184

Recommended reading 184

Resources I used for research 185

Useful websites 201

Introductions
About the author:

My name is Eleanor Worsley. In 2014 I received a diagnosis of Bipolar Type Two after five years of having a Major Depressive Disorder diagnosis. I turn 28 years old on 13th July 2018. I live with my parents in Plymouth, Devon because the last few times I lived on my own I ended up very poorly indeed and tried to take my own life.

I have definitely experienced bipolar symptoms since Sixth Form, but there is no history of bipolar in my family, so we weren't looking out for anything.

In 2009 I went to university and studied Ancient History. Despite being overwhelmingly ill during my first year I managed to work hard enough to scrape a First Class overall. I'm still so proud of this. After university I worked a series of temporary jobs for a year, including several Teaching Assistant positions. In 2013 I began Initial Teacher Training to become a history teacher. I became severely depressed part way through and took three months longer than my colleagues to finish my training but came out with Distinctions across the board. Again, I am really proud of this.

I received my BPII diagnosis at the end of my teacher training when a psychiatrist clocked that for me everything was either amazing or catastrophically awful. I had been experiencing periods of hypomania and severe depression for years and no one had noticed. Finally, I knew what was up with me, why I felt and seemed so different to everyone else.

Now, I am in therapy, I see a Community Psychiatric Nurse once a week, attend a bipolar support group fortnightly and see a psychiatrist every three months (usually). I got really, really ill again in 2015, and I am still recovering.

About the book:

When I was first diagnosed with bipolar disorder type two (BPII) I decided I wanted to know as much about my disorder as possible, so I started reading and haven't really stopped since. In all my reading and research, I have only found three books dedicated to BPII: one information book, one self-help book, and one autobiography; all American. There are a few journal and magazine articles, but most people don't get to reading those. In my opinion just three books are no where near enough, that was my motivation for writing this book dedicated to BPII.

'Life with Bipolar Type Two' has a twofold purpose: one, to educate and inform, two, to guide and support. Most sections are a combination of information and self-help, some are just one or the other. But I have tried to only include that which is relevant to people with BPII.

This book is predominantly designed for people with a BPII diagnosis, but I hope it will also prove useful to loved ones and healthcare professionals who choose to read it. Often, I use the terms 'we' and 'us' because I am very much including myself in the BPII crowd and some of what I've written I only learnt whilst researching for the book.

'Life with Bipolar Type Two' is broken down into five main chapters, each with several short sections for each topic relevant to the chapter title. I've written it this way because when people with BPII are hypomanic or depressed we often have very poor concentration, so reading a short snippet rather than a long chapter is more manageable and digestible.

The chapters of the book are as follows:

Chapter One is 'Bipolar in General'. In this chapter we explore what bipolar disorder and in particular BPII is and how it is diagnosed. Sections include; 'What causes bipolar disorder?', 'Misdiagnosis' and 'History of Bipolar'.

Chapter Two is 'Symptoms', where we discuss the symptoms of BPII. Sections include; 'Depression', 'Self-harm' and 'Sex and Hypersexuality'.

Chapter Three is 'Treatment'. In this section we look at psychiatry, psychotherapy, medications and therapies used to treat BPII.

Chapter Four is 'Management and Lifestyle'. Here we elaborate on some lifestyle choices and coping mechanisms we can use to manage our lives with BPII. Sections include; 'Mindfulness', 'Stress' and 'Sleep'.

Chapter Five is a collection of short essays entitled 'My Musings'. In this chapter we cover some other relevant ideas related to BPII and some of my opinions. Topics include; 'Bipolar: friend or foe?', 'A reason, not an excuse' and 'My bipolar idols'.

Throughout the book I refer to the DSM-IV (Diagnostic and Statistical Manual of Mental Disorders) which is essentially the diagnostic bible for psychiatrists.

I hope you find this book as useful to read as I found it to write.

Chapter One:

Bipolar in General

What is Bipolar Disorder?

Previously known as manic depression,[1] bipolar disorder is a mental health condition known as a mood disorder, or affective disorder, characterised by extreme shifts in mood between high (mania) and low (depression).[2] The shifts in mood in bipolar are distinctly episodic or cyclic,[3] though mood states may last for several months or even years. Mood states range from mania (extreme high) to melancholia/major depression (extreme low), with hypomania (mild high), dysthymia (mild low) and euthymia (normal mood) in between. These moods are each characterised by a range of symptoms, though the symptoms vary from person to person and even from episode to episode.[4]

Typically, affective disorders are diagnosed by a psychiatrist not a GP, who will use criteria from the DSM-IV to diagnose, so if you're not sure whether you have bipolar disorder type two (or any mental health condition) explain to your GP and ask to be referred to a psychiatrist. To receive a diagnosis of bipolar disorder someone must have suffered at least one major depressive episode and at least one either manic or hypomanic episode.

Bipolar disorder is estimated to affect between 1% and 5% of the general population,[5] with somewhere between 60 million[6] and 250 million[7] people living with bipolar worldwide and approximately one

---

[1] NIMH, 2018; Fletcher, 2017; NHS, 2016; NICE, 2014:6; Hodges, 2012:13; Kennard, 2011:2; Marohn, 2011:3; Haycock, 2010:1; Evans & Allen, 2009:151; Suppes & Keck, 2005:1.1; Duke & Hochman, 1993:32.
[2] NIMH, 2018; APA, 2017; MacGill, 2016; NHS, 2016; Marohn, 2011:3; Evans & Allen, 2009:151-152; Miller, 2009:233; Frank et al., 2006; NCCMH, 2006:70; Suppes & Keck, 2005:1.1; Perry et al., 1999; Zaretsky et al., 1999; Duke & Hochman, 1993:xxiv.
[3] Mehta, 2016.
[4] Evans & Allen, 2009;152; Mondimore, 1999:1.
[5] Fletcher, 2017; Sandiou, 2017; NHS, 2016; NICE, 2014:6; Hodges, 2012:11; Marohn, 2011:4; Guyol, 2006:1; Suppes & Keck, 2005:2.1; Zaretsky et al., 1999; Jamison, 1997; Duke & Hochman, 1993:44.
[6] Sandiou, 2017; Mehta, 2016.
[7] Haycock, 2010:1.

million in the UK alone.[8] And up to 46% of people who experience an episode of depression will later have a manic or hypomanic episode and be rediagnosed with bipolar disorder.[9]

According to Miklowitz and colleagues, bipolar disorder is the sixth leading cause of disability worldwide.[10] In a 2005 report it was decided that of the sample group, 82.9% of those with bipolar disorder (types one and two) were deemed to be serious risk, 17.1% deemed to be of moderate risk, and 0% deemed mild or no risk,[11] meaning bipolar should be classed as a moderate to severe disorder.

Bipolar disorder has a high rate of 'morbidity' and 'mortality'[12] and is one of the world's leading causes of suicide. Those with bipolar have a 15% greater chance of dying by suicide than the rest of the general population[13] and as many as one in five people with bipolar will commit suicide.[14]

Bipolar Type I disorder affects men and women equally.[15]

According to the DSM-IV there are three main subtypes of bipolar disorder: Bipolar Type One Disorder (BPI), Bipolar Type Two Disorder (BPII), and Cyclothymia. The main difference in the DSM's three diagnoses is one of 'degree' or severity of symptoms.[16] In most statistics either only BPI, or BPI & BPII are considered. Rarely does cyclothymia or Bipolar Not-Otherwise-Specified (BP-NOS) feature. Though some researchers try to use the full 'bipolar

---

[8] bipolarUK, 2018.
[9] NCCMH, 2006:99.
[10] Miklowitz et al., 2007a.
[11] Kessler et al., 2005.
[12] Bauer et al, 2006; NCCMH, 2006:102; Zaretsky et al., 1999; Jamison, 1997.
[13] Guyol, 2006:1-2.
[14] Marohn, 2011:4; Jamison, 1997.
[15] Marohn, 2011:4; Evans & Allen, 2009:152; Guyol, 2006:1; Jamison, 1997.
[16] Haycock, 2010:8.

spectrum disorders' in their analyses.[17]

The majority of cases of bipolar develop in the late teenage years and early twenties,[18] though some people develop bipolar during childhood or decades later.

Bipolar disorder is considered a chronic[19] and incurable disorder.[20] However it is treatable,[21] and people with bipolar can go on to lead full and productive lives.[22]

What is Bipolar Type Two (BPII)?

Most of the available literature on bipolar disorder focuses on bipolar type one (BPI). A lot of them briefly explain what BPII is, but rarely do they go into detail, and very rarely is it the focus of discussion. This is probably because BPII is often seen as a less severe form of bipolar than BPI. I believe this concept trivialises the nature of the disorder. Though this is nothing compared to the literature's treatment of cyclothymia which barely gets a mention. Unfortunately, cyclothymia is not the purview of this book, but should you wish to gain some insight into what it is like to live with cyclothymia I highly recommend the autobiographies of Stephen Fry.

So, back to BPII: Bipolar type two is diagnosed if a patient presents to a psychiatrist having experienced three mood states: hypomania (mild mania), melancholia (major depression) and euthymia (normal

---

[17] Dunner, 2003.
[18] NICE, 2014:6; Marhon, 2011:4; Evans & Allen, 2009:152; NCCMH, 2006:77; Jamison, 1997.
[19] Bauer et al., 2006.
[20] bipolarUK, 2018; Moezzi, 2016; Guyol, 2006:1.
[21] bipolarUK, 2018; APA, 2017; Fast & Preston, 2012:52; Haycock, 2010:252; NCCMH, 2006:101; Suppes & Keck, 2005:1.1; Mondimore, 1999:48; Jamison, 1997; Duke & Hochman, 1993:xxvi.
[22] APA, 2017; Lamden, 2014; Hodges, 2012:13; NCCMH, 2006:101; Mondimore, 1999:217.

mood).[23] The case history must include a minimum one period of melancholia lasting at least two weeks and having significant impairment on daily functioning, and a minimum of one period of hypomania lasting at least four days.[24] BPII is often more difficult to diagnose than BPI as mania is much more pronounced in effect than hypomania.[25]

In BPII the frequency of depressive episodes in particuar far exceeds that of BPI[26] and in fact we appear to be symptomatic 53.9% of the time; 50.3% in depressive cycles, 1.3% in hypomanic cycles, and 2.3% either rapid cycling or in mixed episodes[27] which is a significant amount of one's life to be having bipolar episodes. On average, episodes of depression in BPII also often last longer than BPI, 52.2 weeks and 24.3 weeks respectively.[28]

There is some evidence that BPII may actually have some 'genetic, clinical and biochemical factors' different from BPI[29] and may in fact be a separate and distinct 'syndrome'.[30]

It has been suggested that, unlike BPI, BPII may affect more women than men.[31]

It is posited that BPII is less severe than BPI[32] and causes less disruption to the sufferer's life,[33] but several 'longitudinal studies have found the bipolar II is far more impairing than [was] once

---

[23] NIMH, 2018; Kennard, 2011:6; Evans & Allen, 2009:153; Fieve, 2006:25; Judd et al., 2003; Mondimore, 1999:39; Duke & Hochman, 1993:37.
[24] Haycock, 2010:9; Evans & Allen, 2009:157; Suppes & Keck, 2005:4.3.
[25] Dunner, 2003.
[26] Fast & Preston, 2012:20; Baek et al., 2011.
[27] Judd et al., 2003.
[28] Mondimore, 1999:40.
[29] Fieve, 2006:x.
[30] Harkavy-Friedman et al., 2006.
[31] Nichols, 2016; NCCMH, 2006:77.
[32] Serretti et al., 2002; Mondimore, 1999:40.
[33] Haycock, 2010:10.

thought'.[34] Even the DSM-IV-TR (Text Revision) states, 'Although Bipolar II is thought to be less severe than Bipolar I in regards to symptom intensity, it is actually more severe and distressing with respect to episode frequency and overall course'.[35] Which makes no illusions as to the fact that '[symptomology] severely fluctuates frequently' in those with BPII.[36] And BPII may actually be more common than BPI[37] affecting between 0.2% and 10.9% of the population.[38] NICE (National Institute for Health and Care Excellence) estimates that 0.4% of the general population has BPII.[39]

Furthermore, BPII has a very high rate of comorbidity (the co-existence of other disorders), especially with anxiety disorders, and substance or alcohol abuse.[40]

What Causes Bipolar Disorder?

Most scientists agree that there is no single cause of bipolar disorder,[41] and certainly no one as yet knows the full cause.[42] To date there are no laboratory tests which can be used to confirm a bipolar diagnosis.[43] There are several hypotheses about the cause(s) of bipolar disorder, but it is generally accepted that bipolar develops as a result of a combination of factors.[44]

Neurochemistry/biochemistry:

There is a lot of evidence supporting that bipolar is linked to, if not

---

[34] Roberts et al., 2013:vii.

[35] Hodges, 2012:15.

[36] Judd et al., 2003.

[37] Mondimore, 1999:40-41.

[38] NCCMH, 2006:77.

[39] NICE, 2014:6.

[40] Roberts et al, 2013:vii; Mondimore, 1999:40.

[41] NIMH, 2018; NCCMH, 2006:80; Suppes & Keck, 2005:1.2.

[42] NHS, 2016; White, 2014:11; Marohn, 2011:25; Guyol, 2006:12.

[43] Mondimore, 1999:29; Duke & Hochman, 1993:31.

[44] NCCMH, 2006:375; Duke & Hochman, 1993:81 & 115.

caused by, 'problems with the brain's chemical messengers',[45] more usually known as neurotransmitters. The functioning and/or levels of neurotransmitters (in particular serotonin, noradrenaline and dopamine) could account for mood swings.[46] 'The success of drugs that affect neurotransmitter levels in treating mood disorders supports the theory that these illnesses have biological roots'.[47]

Genetics:

Of all factors contributing to bipolar, family history is the strongest indicator.[48] Francis Mondimore actually calls a family history of affective disorders a 'red flag for a mood disorder diagnosis'.[49] It appears there is a 'genetic vulnerability' factor to bipolar disorder.[50] Somewhere between 66% and 90% of individuals with bipolar have at least one relative with bipolar or another affective disorder, like unipolar depression or schizo-affective disorder.[51] If one of your parents or siblings has bipolar you are 2-10 times more likely to develop the disorder yourself depending on the study;[52] that being said, two thirds of children with a bipolar parent never develop bipolar.[53] There is significant evidence that BPII runs in families: 40% of the first-degree relatives of someone with BPII will also have BPII, and 22% of first-degree relatives of someone with BPI will also have BPII.[54] This all contributes to the theory that BPII has a genetic component.

---

[45] Roberts et al, 2013:15; Evans & Allen, 2009:151 & 154; Owen & Saunders, 2008:17; Duke & Hochman, 1993:xxvi.
[46] Sandiou, 2017; NHS, 2016; Railton, 2016; White, 2014:11; Marohn, 2011:44-45; Haycock, 2010:59; Miller, 2009:233; Fieve, 2006:33-34.
[47] Evans & Allen, 2009:151.
[48] Haycock, 2010:47; Miller, 2009:237; Mondimore, 1999:191.
[49] Mondimore, 1999:38.
[50] NIMH, 2018; Sandiou, 2017; NHS, 2016; Nichols, 2016; White, 2014:27; Marohn, 2011:25; Haycock, 2010:23; NCCMH, 2006:80; Fieve, 2006:66; Mondimore, 1999:29.
[51] APA, 2017; Evans & Allen, 2009:150; Owen & Saunders, 2008:36; NCCMH, 2006:102; Suppes & Keck, 2005:2.4; Mondimore, 1999:195.
[52] Haycock, 2010:60; Evans & Allen, 2009:154; Duke & Hochman, 1993:81.
[53] Haycock, 2010:60.
[54] Fieve, 2006:66; Mondimore, 1999:41.

Physiology:

Various 'brain imaging techniques have found differences in the brains of people with bipolar disorder and those without'.[55] CT and MRI scans show differences in brain regions associated with processing emotions and in controlling emotional reactions.[56] Many of these differences are in the limbic system. And though not all studies agree, 'several have detected decreased volume in... the striatum and amygdala', both regions strongly associated with emotions and mood.[57] Also, fMRI, SPECT and PET scans, which indicate brain cell activity, have shown that brain cell activity 'decreases with depression and increases with mania'.[58] So physiology may play a role.

Environment:

It is very important to note the role of environment in the onset, if not the general development, of bipolar.[59] It is apparent that environmental factors trigger the onset of bipolar symptoms, both in the first instance and for many proceeding episodes. We know this because symptoms usually begin after a particularly stressful event, situation or change.[60] It is now generally accepted that environmental factors can alter the structure of our brains and impact mood.[61] So although environment alone may not cause BPII, it does at least have a part in the development of BP episodes.

Age of onset:

---

[55] White, 2014:11.
[56] NIMH, 2018; Mondimore, 1999:29.
[57] Haycock, 2010:57-58.
[58] Haycock, 2010:58-59.
[59] NHS, 2016; White, 2014:27; NCCMH, 2006:375.
[60] APA, 2017; Mehta, 2016; NHS, 2016; Nichols, 2016; White, 2014:27; Haycock, 2010:63; Evans & Allen, 2009:154; Miller, 2009:237; Suppes & Keck, 2005:2.6; Mondimore, 1999:223.
[61] Owen & Saunders, 2008:36-37.

Symptoms of bipolar disorder usually first develop in the late teens and early twenties.[62] Though some people show signs of bipolar disorder from early childhood, and others don't develop the disorder until much later in life.

History of Bipolar:

Bipolar disorder has been explored in various forms for over two millennia. Here is a rough timeline I have created from various sources.[63]

Date	Event
BC 2000	Written accounts of mood disorders from Egypt
BC 500	Several Greek and Persian physicians made connections between mania and melancholia
BC 300	Hippocrates describes the four humours and links them to psychiatric disorders
AD 100	Soranus of Ephesus describes a remitting illness of mania and depression
150	Aretaius of Cappadocia 'melancholia is without any doubt the beginning and even part of the disorder called mania'
625-690	Paul of Aegina links mania and melancholia together as one illness
Medieval	Psychiatric disorders put down to witch craft and

---

[62] MacGill, 2016; Mehta, 2016; NHS, 2016; Nichols, 2016; Railton, 2016; Kennard, 2011:2; Marohn, 2011:4; Miklowitz et al, 2008; Suppes & Keck, 2005:1.1; Mondimore, 1999:225.

[63] Marohn, 2011:15-16; Haycock, 2010:7-8; Owen & Saunders, 2008:17-18; Fieve, 2006:14 & 39; NCCMH, 2006:70 & 100-101; Suppes & Keck, 2005:1.4-1.5; Mondimore, 1999:1, 55, 61-63 & 68; Duke & Hochman, 1993:xxvi.

Life With Bipolar Type Two

period	demonic possession
1650	Richard Burton writes a book on melancholia and mentions mania too
1705-1776	Robert James in England connected mania and melancholia saying they were caused by 'Congestion of Blood in the Brain'
1851	Jean-Pierre Falret coined the term 'la folie circulaire' (circular madness) describing mania and depression as part of the same illness
1854	Jules Baillarger coined the term 'la folie à double forme' (madness of two forms) which did not recognise the symptom-free periods
1877	Hecker described 'partial mental disorder', later cyclothymia
1896	Emil Kraeplin first coined the term manic depression
1899	Emil Kraeplin solidified the concept of manic-depression, suggesting that all mood disorders were part of a continuum, and made it clear that mood disorders were not rare
1900	Wernicke asserts that bipolar is distinct from depression
1911	Karl Kleist distinguishes manic-depression from unipolar depression
1920s	Sigmund Freud believed mental illness was caused by psychological factors

1949	John Cade in Australia was convinced that bipolar was a biological not psychological illness
1953	Term "bipolar" coined by Karl Kleist in Germany
1958	DSM-I included manic depression as a legitimate illness
1966	Angst & Perris independently characterised bipolar as different from unipolar depression in 'clinical presentation, evolution, family history and therapeutic response'
1968	DSM-II changed the term from manic depression to manic-depressive psychosis, wherein people oscillate between mania and depression
1976	Dunner et al. differentiate between BPI and BPII
1980	American Psychiatric Association renamed manic depression as bipolar disorder to reflect the 'bi-polarity' of the condition
1980	DSM-III changed the term from manic-depressive psychosis to bipolar affective disorder
1994	DSM-IV subdivided bipolar affective disorder into Bipolar I Disorder and Bipolar II Disorder, along with detailing the differences
late 1990s	Care of people with BP was now mostly psychiatric outpatient and inpatient services, 50% had contact with Community Mental Health Teams, few were treated in hospitals or lived in supported accommodation, Psychoeducation was not widely

	provided
1996	Akiskal sees bipolar as a spectrum, suggesting BPIII and further subcategories for BPI and BPII

Diagnosis:

If anyone thinks they have bipolar type two disorder, the first step is to go to their GP.[64] If you have a list of symptoms matching the depressive and hypomanic descriptions given in this book, then they should be willing to make a referral to psychiatric services for a mental health assessment. You have taken the first step to getting help, this is more than 50% of people with psychiatric conditions ever do.[65] If it turns out that you do have BPII, don't worry, you have a very manageable condition.[66] Bipolar can't be cured, but it can be managed.[67]

The American Foundation for Suicide Prevention suggests 80%-90% of bipolar cases 'can be treated effectively'.[68] BP is quite manageable with the right combination of medication and psychotherapy.[69] It can take years to find the right combination of treatments, but it usually does happen.[70] And it is important to know that most 'people … can receive most of their treatment without having to stay in a hospital'; sectioning is usually reserved for if you become a danger to yourself or others,[71] or become psychotic.

Your new psychiatrist should ensure you are well informed about

---

[64] NIMH, 2018.
[65] Kessler et al., 2005.
[66] Fast & Preston, 2012:52.
[67] Owen & Saunders, 2008:57.
[68] Fast, 2006.
[69] NHS, 2016; Fieve, 2006:xi.
[70] McManamy, 2006:8.
[71] NHS, 2016.

every step of the assessment and involve you in any decisions made about the outset of treatment.[72] You will probably be encouraged to invite a family member or carer to your first appointment, so they can corroborate your history and help you recall what is covered in the meeting. And the assessment should be tailored to you, just as your initial treatment and care plan should be tailored to you.[73] When discussing the development of your initial treatment and care plan, your psychiatrist should not only discuss meds, but also psychological interventions and self-management.[74]

Misdiagnosis:

Diagnosing mood disorders is a lengthy process fraught with challenges, especially for BPII. Initial misdiagnosis of BPII patients is very common; 69% or 70% of people with bipolar are misdiagnosed on their first visit with a mental health professional.[75] Because of the crossover of symptoms, often people with bipolar disorder are misdiagnosed with borderline personality disorder, unipolar depression,[76] or schizophrenia,[77] and even chronic fatigue.[78] In fact, 9% of those diagnosed with Major Depressive Disorder go on to be rediagnosed as BPII.[79] Also because so many people with bipolar are initially misdiagnosed, some experts believe the rates of people with bipolar disorder are actually much higher than statistics currently suggest.[80]

Difficulties with diagnosis arise from: firstly, the fact that we tend to go see a doctor when we're depressed, not when we're happy;[81]

---

[72] NICE, 2014:19-20.
[73] Marohn, 2011:27.
[74] Yatham et al., 2005.
[75] Owen & Saunders, 2008:46; McManamy, 2006:43.
[76] Nichols, 2016; Mehta, 2016; Jackel, 2010; Owen & Saunders, 2008:47; Duke & Hochman, 1993:45.
[77] NIMH, 2018; Owen & Saunders, 2008:49; Duke & Hochman, 1993:45.
[78] Evans & Saunders, 2008:49.
[79] Mondimore, 1999:40.
[80] Duke & Hochman, 1993:xxiv.
[81] NIMH, 2018.

secondly, BPII shares a lot of symptoms with borderline personality disorder and schizophrenia (though both of those are consistent not episodic); and thirdly, hypomania is notoriously difficult to diagnose[82] because we as patients simply don't think to mention those times when we are in our best moods. And finally, there is no simple test,[83] instead psychiatrists have to be on the ball and ask about history of mood, episodes of overactivity, other episodic and sustained changes in behaviour and activity levels, symptoms between episodes, triggers and patterns of mood episodes and family history, before they even start on your current symptoms, social and occupational functioning or assess for comorbidities (co-existing disorders).[84]

Because of the problems with diagnosis, and the fact that some people just don't seek help[85] until they have no choice, the average time between onset of symptoms and correct diagnosis and treatment is between eight and ten years[86] and takes an average of four doctors.[87] This is a really long time, but it is unfortunately the norm. This decade of waiting, misdiagnosis and possible mis-treatment is not only inconvenient, it can be painful or even dangerous. People can be given the wrong treatment, making their symptoms worse or even introducing new symptoms. People may not receive any type of formal diagnosis until they end up in A&E or a jail cell at a police station; by then damage has already been done.

Unfortunately for a lot of people with BPII things have to get a lot better before they get better. What I mean is, some people have to turn up at the GP surgery or psychiatrist's clinic after months of depression and be high as a kite before it is realised they have

---

[82] Dunner, 2003.
[83] Owen & Saunders, 2008:46-47.
[84] NICE, 2014:19.
[85] NCCMH, 2006:101.
[86] NICE, 2014:6; Hodges, 2012:11; Kennard, 2011:3; Marohn, 2011:5; Owen & Saunders, 2008:46; Fieve, 2006:27; Mondimore, 1999:40.
[87] Owen & Saunders, 2008:46-47.

hypomania.

Children Whose Parents Have Bipolar Disorder:
A fair amount of research has been conducted looking at the heredity of bipolar. It comes with some interesting and perhaps surprising results.

First of all, not all children with a bipolar parent will develop bipolar disorder;[88] in fact two thirds do not.[89] However, having one bipolar parent puts a child at a 10%-30% chance of developing the disorder,[90] and having two bipolar parents increases that chance as high as 75%.[91] If you have a parent with bipolar disorder you have a twenty-something percent chance of developing a different affective disorder.[92]

We know genetics plays a part, but does childhood environment play a part as well?

Less work has been done on how having a bipolar parent may impact a child's homelife and childhood in general.

Some research shows that having a parent with bipolar can lead to a more disrupted childhood.[93] This might be due to several possible factors: parental sexual indiscretions, financial troubles, the parent having 'wide and unpredictable mood swings', and drug abuse or alcoholism.[94] Chang and colleagues found that families 'with a bipolar parent differ from the average family in having less cohesion and organization, and more conflict'.[95] That is not to say that people with BP necessarily make bad parents, it simply seems to be the

---

[88] Fieve, 2006:67.
[89] Haycock, 2010:60.
[90] Mondimore, 1999:195.
[91] Marohn, 2011:5.
[92] Mondimore, 1999:195.
[93] Leader, 2013:27.
[94] Fieve, 2006:67.
[95] Chang et al., 2002.

case that having a bipolar parent can result in a more erratic, and perhaps more interesting, upbringing for any children born into the family. The impacts, though they may seem negative at the time, can have positive benefits in the long term, such as a much stronger sense of empathy and a greater ease in identifying other people's moods.

So, a genetic predisposition and possibly a disrupted childhood could both contribute to the development of bipolar disorder. In fact, 'between 13% and 28%' develop bipolar before they are thirteen years old.[96] It is worth noting that 10% of teenagers with recurrent depression will go on to have bipolar disorder.[97]

Medical Conditions that Mimic BP Symptomology

As if diagnosing bipolar wasn't difficult enough, there are also a plethora of medical conditions which have some of the same symptoms as the disorder.[98]

Just some of the conditions that mimic bipolar symptoms are:[99]

- Hypo- and hyperthyroidism
- Dementia
- Parkinson's Disease
- Huntington's Disease
- Cerebrovascular diseases, including stroke
- Lupus
- Some viral infections, including HIV
- Pancreatic cancer
- Multiple sclerosis
- Lyme disease
- Syphilis.

---

[96] Miklowitz et al., 2008.
[97] Hodges, 2012:11.
[98] Fieve, 2006:162.
[99] Marohn, 2011:47; Fieve, 2006:162; NCCMH, 2006:13.

Bipolar-type symptoms can also present if a person has a vitamin B_{12} deficiency[100] or if they have an adverse reaction to corticosteroids used to treat inflammatory conditions.[101]

---

[100] Marohn, 2011:47.
[101] Fieve, 2006:163.

Chapter Two:

Symptoms

Depression

I've decided to give you the section on depression before anything else. This is because people with BPII spend around half of their time depressed,[102] so it's a big issue to discuss.

Along with hypomania, depression is one of the hallmarks of BPII. Depression can be very basically characterised as low mood, low energy, low motivation, low pleasure, too much sleep and too many carbs; at least in my experience and from talking to others with bipolar disorder.

The Oxford English Dictionary defines depression thus:

'depression, n. 1. Severe despondency and dejection, especially when long-lasting.'

But that doesn't quite cover it... Depression is a broad and varied diagnosis;[103] it covers a spectrum of sadness and a wide collection of symptoms.

Bipolar depression is difficult to say the least. And the worst of it is, most people with BPII spend around half their life depressed.[104] People with bipolar spend a 'whopping 40:1' ratio spent in depression versus hypomania and mania.[105] And on average depressive episodes are longer than manic or hypomanic episodes.[106]

There are levels of depression recognised by the DSM-IV: Depression can be classified as subsyndromal (some symptoms but not enough or with enough impairment to qualify for diagnosis), mild (some symptoms with mild impact on daily functioning), moderate (several symptoms with moderate impact on daily functioning) and severe (many symptoms with significant impact on

---

[102] NCCMH, 2006:71.
[103] NICE, 2009:6.
[104] Fieve, 2006:57; McManamy, 2006:71; Judd et al., 2003.
[105] Jackel, 2010; NCCMH, 2006:281.
[106] NCCMH, 2006:245.

daily functioning),[107] and compared to unipolar depression bipolar depression is much more variable in its symptom severity.[108] That being said major bipolar depressive episodes are very similar to major unipolar depressive episodes,[109] so reading books about depression may be helpful to those with BPII. Though bipolar depression is more likely to have 'atypical' features like sleeping a lot.[110] Subsyndromal depressive symptoms between mood episodes are common for people with BPII and is a cause of significant interpersonal and occupational disability.[111] Also, 10%-18% of people who experience a mild depression will go on to develop major depression within a year.[112]

Symptoms:

The DSM-IV states that to qualify diagnostically as depressed you must have substantially low mood and exhibit at least four of its depression symptoms for a minimum of two weeks,[113] with a marked impact on your daily functioning.

Here is a list of the DSM's depression diagnostic criteria:

- Insomnia or hypersomnia (inability to/difficulty with sleeping, or an excessive need to sleep.
- Significant increase or decrease in appetite.
- Inexplicable or unfounded feelings of guilt.
- Feelings of worthlessness.
- Decreased energy levels, lethargy.
- Inability to focus or concentrate.
- Thoughts of, or actions taken towards suicide.

---

[107] Chellingsworth & Farrand, 2015:39.
[108] NCCMH, 2006:98.
[109] NCCMH, 2006:71.
[110] McManamy, 2006:70.
[111] NCCMH, 2006:72.
[112] Suppes & Keck, 2005:3.9.
[113] Roberts et al., 2013:8; Khamba et al., 2011; Jamison, 1997.

Again, I don't think it quite covers it. So here is a more comprehensive list of my own compilation, based on my experiences with depression and extensive research: [114]

- All the DSM criteria, plus:
- Lack of interest or pleasure in activities previously found enjoyable (anhedonia).
- Withdrawal from social interaction.
- Feelings of deep sadness.
- Persistent aches or pains with no clear explanation.
- Psychotic symptoms such as hallucinations.
- Paranoia.
- Irritability.
- Anxiety.
- Lack of self-care/personal hygiene.
- Emotional numbness.
- Feelings of emptiness.
- An inability to do day-to-day tasks like laundry or getting out of bed.
- Lack of motivation.
- Feelings of "loss of self" or becoming a "shell".
- Compulsions to, or actions of self-harm.
- Negative self-thoughts/self-image.
- Tearfulness.
- Indecisiveness.
- Catatonia (staring into space, doing nothing).
- Loss of libido.
- Poor memory.
- Slowed thinking.

---

[114] NIMH, 2018; APA, 2017; Fletcher, 2017; MacGill, 2016; Mehta 2016; NHS, 2016; Chellingsworth & Farrand, 2015:36 & 38-39; Roberts et al., 2013:8 & 44-45; Shabbir et al., 2013; Fast & Preston, 2012:21; Hodges, 2012:15 & 29; ; Kennard, 2011:4; Khamba et al., 2011; Marohn, 2011:4&9-10; Haycock, 2010:5-6; Jackel, 2010; Evans & Allen, 2009:155; Miller, 2009:61-62; Brugue et al., 2008; Owen & Saunders, 2008:22; Fieve, 2006:47; Guyol, 2006:5-6; NCCMH, 2006:71; Suppes & Keck, 2005:3.9-3.11; Mondimore, 1999:18; Jamison, 1997; Duke & Hochman, 1993:xxv.

- Psychomotor retardation (slow physical movements).

Though these are not DSM criteria for depression, if you go to a GP or psychiatrist with several of these symptoms having a marked impact on your ability to function in daily life, they may very well diagnose you as depressed.

The effects of these symptoms can be mild, moderate or severe, as described above. In all its forms depression can be disruptive and in its more severe forms depression can devastate lives.[115] It can find us 'rehashing [our] failings, guilt, or issues' in unhealthy and destructive ways.[116] Depression is a horrible place to be.[117] And depression accounts for a high proportion of the disability, morbidity and suicide rates of BPII.[118] It has possibly the most significant effect on quality of life out of all bipolar mood states and symptoms;[119] we feel guilty about everything,[120] nothing is of interest to us,[121] we repeat ourselves endlessly,[122] we may feel irritable constantly,[123] we cry uncontrollably,[124] we are exhausted all the time,[125] and we think in negative ways about everything.[126]

What does depression feel like?

In my personal experience there are four main states of depression, though there are subtypes:

1. Numb and vacant: where we just sit and stare at the wall for hours; when nothing happens, we do nothing, and

---

[115] Jackel, 2010.
[116] Wooldridge, 2016:169.
[117] Hodges, 2012:29.
[118] Thase & Sachs, 2000; Zaretsky et al., 1999.
[119] Vojta et al., 2001.
[120] Khamba et al., 2011.
[121] Fast, 2006.
[122] Leader, 2013:18.
[123] Deckersbach, 2004.
[124] Haycock, 2010:171.
[125] Roberts et al., 2013:41.
[126] Roberts et al., 2013:61.

nothing is of interest.[127] Sometimes this state is described as being catatonic.
2. Self-loathing and angry: where we hate ourselves for every little thing we do or do not do. Where we constantly beat ourselves up for feeling depressed and everything just makes us more angry and irritable.[128]
3. Ruminating: where we dwell on past mistakes, missteps and losses. Where our brain takes over and we cannot focus on anything except our wandering minds.[129]
4. Weepy: where we just cry. Where we cry for every reason and no reason at all. We just cry uncontrollably.[130] And we are miserable all the time.

Causes and triggers:

The main biological cause for depression seems to be a decrease in the activity of several neurotransmitters in the brain, in particular dopamine and serotonin.[131]

Environmental triggers also play a part. A trigger is any event or situation which directly leads to a mood episode. 'When severe negative life events occur', such as natural disaster,[132] job loss or marital breakdown, 'they appear to trigger increases in bipolar depression'.[133]

However, in many cases, there does not need to be an external trigger for depression, it could just be part of your natural cycle, or it could be a combination of smaller stresses.[134]

Treatment and management:

---

[127] Fast, 2006.
[128] Dunner, 2003.
[129] Wooldridge, 2016:169.
[130] Haycock, 2010:171.
[131] White, 2014:70; Fieve, 2006:119.
[132] Nolen-Hoeksema & Morrow, 1991.
[133] Johnson, 1990.
[134] Todd, 2016:38; Johnson, 1990.

Bipolar depression 'represents a major challenge for treating clinicians'[135] and we still 'need to develop more effective treatments for bipolar depression',[136] but most episodes of bipolar depression respond well to treatment combinations of medication and psychotherapy.[137]

In terms of medication, there are mood stabilisers and antidepressants; a combination of which is typically prescribed for bipolar depression (more about meds later).[138] There is also psychotherapy (more about psychological interventions later).[139]

> If you ever feel suicidal the NHS advice is that you go to A&E.[140] To be honest everyone's best advice is to go to A&E.

Managing depression:

Managing depression is often a long and painful process, but it does happen. Every depressive episode we have ends, eventually. However, there are a lot of things we can do to help speed up the process. Here is a list of examples based my research and experience:[141]

- Take your medications as prescribed (more later).
- Get some gentle exercise; go for a walk (more later).
- Socialise.
- Get in the sunlight.
- Listen to music, anything that makes you feel relaxed or happy.
- Avoid stimulants like caffeine and depressants like alcohol.

---

[135] Thase & Sachs, 2000.
[136] Hlastala et al., 1997.
[137] Fieve, 2006:26.
[138] NICE, 2014:24; NCCMH, 2006:19; Thase & Sachs, 2000.
[139] NICE, 2014;23.
[140] NHS, 2016.
[141] Chellingsworth & Farrand, 2015:55-116; Hodges, 2012:34-35; Miller, 2009:162-169 & 172-179; NCCMH, 2006:293.

- Eat foods that bring back good memories.
- Speak positively to yourself (positive self-talk), compliment yourself, congratulate yourself when you do something difficult or new.
- Go to Cognitive Behavioural Therapy (more later) or get a self-help book.
- Have a massage.
- Keep busy with a structured day.
- Talk to people, tell them how you feel.
- Get a hug, hold someone's hand, gentle human contact is good.
- Stroke an animal, pets are great for us (more later).
- Tackle simpler/less daunting tasks first.
- Keep planned activities in place.
- Change your behaviour in order to change your thoughts (do everything else in the list and you will find that your thoughts and emotions begin to become more positive and relaxed).

Hypomania
What is hypomania?

In 1881, German psychiatrist Mendel coined the term hypomanic to describe the state 'of mild euphoria and hyperactivity' that doesn't progress to 'full-blown mania'.[142] The word hypomania literally means "below or less than mania" and is still used today. Hypomania is sometimes described as being "high" or "up", because of the accompanying euphoria (despite the fact that sometimes hypomania is agitated and irritable more than elated). Hypomania is a state of 'expansive, elevated or agitated mood' that is similar to mania but 'less intense and lacks psychotic symptoms',[143] it is often described as 'euphoria',[144] though when you are irritable and

---
[142] Mondimore, 1999:15.
[143] Evans & Allen, 2009:153.
[144] Roberts et al., 2013:104.

agitated it is not a terribly happy place to be. In order to be diagnosed as hypomania the episode must last at least four days.[145]

Hypomania is the key feature of BPII; if you experience mania it's probably BPI, if you experience no highs at all it's probably Major Depressive Disorder. (Without mania or hypomania it simply isn't bipolar disorder.)[146] As with depressive episodes, hypomania is often triggered by a life event, which may be as simple as receiving praise at work.[147] In hypomania, unlike with mania, normal day-to-day functioning is not usually impaired; in fact 'a person with hypomania can put their extra energy, creativity and mild euphoria' to good use.[148] Mania, and to some extent hypomania, is 'liquid confidence'[149] making a person much more likely to be extroverted and take risks; this can be great or really bad. When hypo, BPIIs are the life and soul of the party, but their constant energy can make them really difficult to live with.[150]

Scientists believe that hypomania, like depression, may be linked to our neurotransmitters, it's also dopamine and serotonin.[151] It is thought that increased activity of these "feel-good" chemicals is what may cause hypomania.

Hypomania in General:

People with BPII are hypomanic an average 1% of the time.[152] That doesn't seem like a lot, but even this much can have a dramatic impact on our lives.

'It is easy for those with Bipolar II to romanticize the hypomanic mood until they experience compulsive gambling or financial loss, impulsivity, hypersexuality, or substance addiction – all behaviours

---

[145] Roberts et al., 2013:8.
[146] NCCMH, 2006:70.
[147] NCCMH, 2006:376.
[148] Owen & Saunders, 2008:25.
[149] Fisher, 2008:128.
[150] Duke & Hochman, 1993:39.
[151] Fieve, 2006:119.
[152] Owen & Saunders, 2008:24; McManamy, 2006:71; NCCMH, 2006:73.

commonly found in those with Bipolar II'.[153] The impulsive nature of hypomania can have 'far-reaching emotional and social consequences'[154] such as divorce, joblessness, bankruptcy, promiscuity and even prison sentences. This and other data collected suggests that 'hypomanic [is a syndrome] characterized by reduced, not increased, sense of well-being and quality of life'.[155]

All that being said and done, hypomania 'may at times be of great benefit' to a person with BPII.[156] Some say that hypomanic 'is a great place to be on the spectrum of the disorder' because productivity, creativity and the ability to communicate 'increases by more than 75% in most people'.[157]

However, a word of caution: 'hypomania can signal a worsening course of illness'.[158] It is not uncommon for those of us with BPII to "crash" out of a hypomania into a severe depression,[159] especially if untreated. This is obviously very dangerous as the depression may be exasperated by sadness at having lost the hypo (short for hypomania), causing a "double-depression" where you become depressed about being depressed.

Hypo vs Mania:

Hypomania is sometimes described as 'mania lite'.[160] The difference between mania and hypomania is the severity of symptoms and severity of impairment, it is a matter 'of degree'.[161] Hypomanias experienced by people with BPII 'are not as impairing' as mania experienced in BPI[162] and some say that hypomania had 'best be thought of as consisting of the symptoms that present at the

---

[153] Fieve, 2006:23-24.
[154] Evans & Allen, 2009:153.
[155] Vojta et al., 2001.
[156] Fieve, 2006:21.
[157] Hodges, 2012:16.
[158] Roberts et al., 2013:112.
[159] NIMH, 2018.
[160] Owen & Saunders, 2008:24.
[161] Fieve, 2006:18.
[162] Roberts et al., 2013:vii.

beginning of a manic episode'.[163] This is because many of the symptoms of mania and hypomania are the same, but they are generally less pronounced in hypomania. Also, while by-and-large mania has a dramatic negative impact on a person's life 'hypomania is a far more productive, active period'[164] and though it may have significant negative impacts upon a person's life, it does not greatly affect daily functioning.

How do you recognise hypomania?

First of all, how do you know hypomania isn't just you being happy that you're not depressed anymore? Well hypomania is recurrent, happiness is not;[165] that is to say, once you've had one hypo episode the rest often look and feel much the same, happiness is short-lived and varies a lot in presentation.

Then there are the symptoms: The DSM-IV lists the following symptoms for hypomania and mania. For it to be hypomania it must be an expansive, elevated or irritable mood, and it must last at least four days, but not have severe impact on daily functioning:

- Not needing or wishing to sleep.
- Rushed/racing thoughts.
- Risk-taking, pleasure-seeking behaviour outside of your normal character (illicit or ill-advised sexual encounters, excessive gambling, spending sprees, dangerous driving).
- Increased distractibility, inability to complete tasks.
- Pressured speech or rushed talking, feeling more talkative than normal.
- Flight of grand ideas.
- Increased goal-oriented activity (at school, work, or in the home).

---

[163] Mondimore, 1999:16.
[164] Fieve, 2006:18.
[165] Duke & Hochman, 1993:39.

However, as with depression, I think this list is far from exhaustive. Based on my own experience and extensive research, here is my more comprehensive list to go on top of the DSM-IV's:[166]

- Markedly increased or decreased appetite.
- Impulsive actions or behaviours.
- Agitation, or an inability to sit still.
- Constantly interrupting or not listening to people.
- Drug or alcohol use that is out of character.
- Either an inability to concentrate or becoming hyper-focused.
- Being quick to anger.
- Inflated self-confidence.
- Feelings of euphoria.
- Grandiosity.
- Hypersexuality.
- Increased creativity.
- Increased productivity.
- Anxiety.

Again, my own list is by no means exhaustive, you may well have your own hypomanic symptoms I have not included. Some of these symptoms may never emerge for you, others may surface when you are in a fully hypo state, others still may appear as prodromes (early warning symptoms). Some of the most typical prodromes or early warning symptoms are lack of sleep, appetite changes and anxiety;[167] these changes may herald an episode and allow you to nip it in the bud.

---

[166] NIMH, 2018; APA, 2017; Fletcher, 2017; bpMagazine, 2016; MacGill, 2016; Mehta, 2016; NHS, 2016; Leader, 2013:38; Roberts et al., 2013:8 & 103; Fast & Preston, 2012:23; Hodges, 2012:13-14; Kennard, 2011:3; Marohn, 2011:3-4; Haycock, 2010:2-5; Evans & Allen, 2009:155-156; Miller, 2009:233-234; Fisher, 2008:114; Owen & Saunders, 2008:26; Fieve, 2006:47; Guyol, 2006:67; McManamy, 2006:64; NCCMH, 2006:74-75; Suppes & Keck, 2005:3.7-3.8; Mondimore, 1999:10; Jamison, 1997; APA, 1994:332; Duke & Hochman, 1993:xxv-xxvi.
[167] Leader, 2013:20.

Life With Bipolar Type Two

Overcoming hypomanic symptoms:

Roberts and colleagues[168] created a list of techniques to overcome impulsivity, which is one of the riskier hypo behaviours. Here are some of their offerings with my own explanations:

- 'The Two-Person Feedback Rule': when you feel the urge to do something you are aware is even mildly out of character, or is uncommon behaviour for you, first ask two different people for their opinion. If both agree that it's a sound, reasonable and safe idea, go ahead. If either one has doubts, don't do it.
- 'Forty-Eight Hour Rule': when you want to do something you know would be an unusual choice for you, wait 48 hours before deciding whether to go ahead; sleep on it twice and if it still seems like a good idea, go ahead with it.
- 'Limit your access to funds': typical hypo behaviours are reckless spending, excessive gambling and risky investments. If you know these behaviours feature in your hypomanias, when you feel a hypomanic episode coming on or your loved ones point out to you that you may be becoming hypomanic, restrict your funds to stop your spending getting out of hand. There are multiple ways you can do this: Many banks will happily set spending limits on your accounts so that you can only withdraw a certain amount each day. Limit your overdraft to a manageable amount; some people live in their overdraft because they have no other choice, but if you can it is best to only have an overdraft of a couple of hundred pounds, or none at all, this way you can't rack up thousands of pounds of debt in a matter of days. Delete all your saved cards from online sites; if you have to enter all your details each time you want to spend online, you are more likely to be considerate about what you spend. Or finally, if you know you get really bad, give your cards to someone you trust (usually a family

---

[168] Roberts et al., 2013:123-124.

member or partner); tell them to allow you to withdraw a limited amount of money each week and you may only have that much, until your hypo subsides. This last one requires a lot of trust, be aware you do not have to give your PIN away, just be supervised when withdrawing cash.
- 'Think before speaking': it may sound trite, but it is important to really think before speaking, texting, calling, emailing, blogging, posting, writing or messaging. Always plan ahead or draft anything important or which might impact you or someone else in a personal or public manner. This way you are less likely to upset or offend and less likely to put your foot in it with important people (like your boss).
- Avoid alcohol and drugs: when we are hypo our inhibitions drop lower than normal. Alcohol and some drugs can exacerbate this leading to risky or inappropriate behaviour. Also, alcohol is a depressant, making it more likely that you will "crash" out of your hypo suddenly, which is dangerous. And drugs like cocaine are stimulants which may emphasise your hypo behaviour making it more extreme, and drugs can easily induce mania and psychosis (even in people with BPII).[169]

To overcome agitation and irritability you should try to engage in relaxing or 'calming activities',[170] like reading, taking a bath, or listening to relaxing, peaceful music (which for you may be anything from whale song to heavy metal, as long as it makes you chill).

To avoid symptoms like changes in appetite or sleep pattern it is important to 'establish a structured routine'.[171] This might include set sleep/wake times where you go to bed at a certain time every night and even if you wake up in the night you stay in bed until a certain time every morning, when your alarm goes off. This should

---

[169] Roberts et al., 2013:123-124.
[170] NCCMH, 2006:393.
[171] NCCMH, 2006:17.

ideally be at the same times each day in order to establish a healthy sleep/wake cycle.

To avoid negative consequences from over-confidence, talkativeness or irritability, you might consider taking some time off work.[172]

Treatment:

There are treatments for hypomania should the 'exuberance [extend] too far into irritability, rage, or poor judgement'.[173]

First of all, if a person develops hypomania whilst on an antidepressant, the antidepressant should be stopped as abruptly as is safe.[174] The same can be said of lamotrigine[175] which should not be continued if a person becomes hypomanic.

In acute hypomania benzodiazepines may be used to calm symptoms,[176] but because they have strong sedative effects and can be addictive, they should only be used in the short term (more about benzodiazepines later). So, in the meantime the hypomanic person should have access and be exposed to 'calming environments and reduced stimulation.[177]

Rapid Cycling

If someone has four or more distinct mood episodes in a 12-month period they are classed as rapid cycling.[178] Between 15% and 20% of people with bipolar disorder experience rapid cycling,[179] with most

---

[172] NCCMH, 2006:393.
[173] Fieve, 2006:26.
[174] NICE, 2014:21; NCCMH, 2006:17.
[175] NICE, 2014:23.
[176] NCCMH, 2006:17.
[177] NICE, 2014:21.
[178] Mehta, 2016; Marohn, 2011:11; Haycock, 2010:16-17; Jackel, 2010; Owen & Saunders, 2008:22; Fieve, 2006:59-60; NCCMH, 2006:76; Mondimore, 1999:50.
[179] Haycock, 2010:17; Jackel, 2010; Evans & Allen, 2009:154; McManamy, 2006:73.

of those being BPII,[180] and especially women.[181] As much as 60% of all people with BP may experience rapid cycling at some point.[182]

Rapid cycling was coined as a term in the 1970s by Drs Fieve & Dunner 'when [they] identified a group of ... patients ... who did not respond well to lithium therapy ... These patients typically had four or more cycles of mania and depression in the 12-month interval prior to lithium treatment'.[183,184] The DSM-IV in 1994, formally adopted the term rapid cycling to define those who experienced four or more mood cycles/states in a year. Rapid cycling is a 'course specifier rather than a specific type of bipolar'[185] meaning that you can have BPI, BPII or Cyclothymia with Rapid Cycling.

Because rapid cycling was not described until the 1970s, some have speculated that it is, in fact, the result of treatment with antidepressants.[186] Now, as a general rule, if a patient presents with rapid cycling all antidepressants are stopped as swiftly as is safely possible.[187]

Another theory is the 'kindling hypothesis', which suggests that over time repeated episodes become more frequent and closer together due to increased sensitisation to triggers.[188] Therefore, the more often you are ill, the more likely you are to become ill in the future, and this trend could be exponential.

Some studies have found that rapid cycling increases depressive symptoms, risk of suicide, causes treatment resistance and is associated with a 'higher incidence of drug misuse'.[189] Other studies have shown no trend toward a greater risk for suicide due to rapid

---

[180] Baek et al., 2011.
[181] Mehta, 2016; Nichols, 2016; Evans & Allen, 2009:154; Fieve, 2006:59; Suppes & Keck, 2005:1.1; Mondimore, 1999:50.
[182] NCCMH, 2006:71.
[183] Fieve, 2006:59-60.
[184] Ghaemi, 2008: Mondimore, 1999:50.
[185] NCCMH, 2006:244.
[186] NHS, 2016; Ghaemi, 2008; Mondimore, 1999:50.
[187] Ghaemi, 2008.
[188] Coryell et al., 2003.
[189] NCCMH, 2006:76; Coryell et al., 2003.

cycling.[190] Certainly rapid cycling makes it more difficult to function in daily life, as you don't know how you're going to feel next week, let alone next month; so making plans is difficult. Especially if you're an ultra-rapid cycler, where you have multiple mood swings possibly even within one day.[191]

There is accumulating evidence that rapid cycling makes bipolar very difficult to treat,[192] as you would imagine; and rapid cycling bipolar may even become completely treatment resistant.

Overall rapid cycling is very difficult to live with and very difficult to manage.

The Stanley Foundation Bipolar Network Survey of 2003 found that people with BPII spend 12% of their time either rapid cycling or in mixed episodes (mixed episodes coming up next).[193]

Mixed Episodes

Mixed episodes, or mixed states, are very much what it says on the tin. A mixed episode (also known as an episode with mixed features, or a mixed mania) is 'a manifestation of bipolar disorder in which depression and mania exist together in one episode'.[194] Essentially the person experiences symptoms at both ends of their spectrum at the same time.[195] For BPII, it is specifically an episode of depression with three or more hypomanic features, or an episode of hypomania with three or more depressive symptoms.[196] It is not uncommon for someone in a mixed episode to feel particularly irritable or paranoid,[197] and very often they present with a similar

---

[190] Wu & Dunner, 1993.
[191] NHS, 2016; Marohn, 2011:11; Evans & Allen, 2009:154; Owen & Saunders, 2008:22; NCCMH, 2006:76.
[192] Ghaemi, 2008; Fieve, 2006:59-60; McManamy, 2006:245; NCCMH, 2006:76.
[193] McManamy, 2006:71.
[194] Marohn, 2011:11.
[195] NIMH, 2018; Mehta, 2016; NHS, 2016; Owen & Saunders, 2008:30-31; Suppes & Keck, 2005:1.3-1.4; Mondimore, 1999:25.
[196] Roberts et al., 2013:9.
[197] Fieve, 2006:159.

mood state as a bipolar depressive[198] with behaviours more commonly associated with hypomania; they may feel depressed and restless at the same time, or feel 'tired but wired'.[199]

It is estimated that approximately two thirds of people with bipolar disorder will experience a mixed state and that those with BPII spend an average 2% of their time in mixed states.[200]

Being in a mixed episode can be very confusing;[201] you don't know if you're up, down or sideways from one minute to the next. You can't make plans because you don't know how you're going to feel in an hour, let alone tomorrow or next week. You can feel despondent but have lots of energy, or you can feel elated but find nothing interests you.

And mixed states can be dangerous.[202] When you are depressed you may well feel suicidal, but not have the energy or motivation to act on it. When you're in a mixed state you may feel suicidal and have an abundance of energy. As such, mixed states put us at a much higher risk of suicide.[203]

Comorbidity

Comorbidity: what is it? Who has it?

Comorbidity, also known as 'dual-diagnosis',[204] means having more than one diagnosis at a time. In psychiatry comorbidity is very common.[205] In one study of people with psychiatric disorders 55% had one diagnosis, 22% had two diagnoses, and 23% had three or more co-existing psychiatric conditions.[206]

---

[198] Vojta et al., 2001.
[199] Owen & Saunders, 2008:30.
[200] Owen & Saunders, 2008:31.
[201] Haycock, 2010:16.
[202] Owen & Saunders, 2008:31.
[203] Jackel, 2010; Owen & Saunders, 2008:31; NCCMH, 2006:22.
[204] Fieve, 2006:120.
[205] Vollebergh, 2001; Krueger, 1999.
[206] Kessler et al., 2005.

With bipolar disorder comorbidity 'is the norm rather than the exception' with about 65% of people with BP suffering with another psychiatric condition at some point in their lives.[207] According to Dr Fieve, comorbid disorders are more common in BPII women than BPII men.[208]

Which comorbidities occur with bipolar?

The most common comorbidities with bipolar are anxiety disorders and substance misuse, 'both of which occur in approximately 30-50% of patients with bipolar disorder'.[209] Other common co-existing disorders are conduct disorders, personality disorders, eating disorders, ADHD and sexual addiction,[210] especially for those with BPII.[211]

Comorbid anxiety disorders:

Comorbid anxiety disorders, such as Generalised Anxiety Disorder (GAD), Obsessive-Compulsive Disorder (OCD) and Panic Disorder are common especially in those of us with BPII.[212] Between 24% and 42% of us have anxiety disorders on top of our bipolar.[213] And there is a much higher incidence of phobia than in the general population.[214]

There is evidence that people who have both BP and anxiety may respond less well to treatment and 'suffer greater functional impairment'.[215] They may also have earlier age at onset of illness, be

---

[207] NIMH, 2018; Fletcher, 2017; Krueger, 2017; Nichols, 2016; Railton, 2016; NICE, 2014:6; Marohn, 2011:5; Evans & Allen, 2009:149; Fieve, 2006:28; NCCMH, 2006:92; Suppes & Keck, 2005:5.13-5.14.
[208] Fieve, 2006:59.
[209] NCCMH, 2006:92.
[210] NICE, 2014:6; Marohn, 2011:5; Suppes & Keck, 2005:5.13-5.14.
[211] Fieve, 2006:28.
[212] NCCMH, 2006:207.
[213] Suppes & Keck, 2005:5.13-5.14.
[214] Baek et al., 2011.
[215] Suppes & Keck, 2005:7.22-7.23.

more likely to have accelerated cycles and be more prone to severe illness and self-harm than those without an anxiety disorder.[216]

For more about anxiety, anxiety disorders and anxiety symptoms, and how to cope, see the section 'Anxiety'.

Comorbid substance misuse:

Many people with bipolar self-medicate with alcohol and/or drugs[217] in fact as many as 61% of people with bipolar have a substance abuse problem, disorder or addiction.[218] This compares with a substance abuse percentage of between 15% and 29% for all those with psychiatric conditions[219] and is five times the prevalence of the general population.[220]

People with BPII are at a higher risk of alcoholism than those with BPI.[221] And substance-related disorders are more common in the families of those with BPII.[222] Also the prevalence rates are significantly higher for those who have both BP and anxiety disorders.[223]

Unfortunately, substance abuse is not only a problem in and of itself that needs to be addressed, usually through psychotherapy,[224] but it also further complicates the course and treatment of the bipolar disorder. Abuse and misuse of substances can trigger bipolar in the first place,[225] it can precipitate depression[226] and mania.[227] People

---

[216] NCCMH, 2006:92.
[217] NHS, 2016; Todd, 2016:15; Marohn, 2011:6; Haycock, 2010:25; Duke & Hochman, 1993:59.
[218] Kennard, 2011:24; Marohn, 2011:56; McManamy, 2006:111; Suppes & Keck, 2005:5.13-5.14; Simon et al., 2004; Mondimore, 1999:170; Duke & Hochman, 1993:59.
[219] Fieve, 2006:119; Regier et al., 1990.
[220] Fieve, 2006:119-120; McManamy, 2006:111.
[221] Mondimore, 1999:40.
[222] Baek et al., 2011.
[223] Simon et al., 2004.
[224] NCCMH, 2006:11.
[225] Owen & Saunders, 2008:37.
[226] APA, 2017; Roberts et al., 2013:52; Marohn, 2011:50; Fieve, 2006:119.
[227] APA, 2017; Marohn, 2011:49-50; Fieve, 2006:120.

with BP and a comorbid substance abuse disorder are more likely to experience mixed episodes or rapid cycling,[228] and are up to 15 times more likely to attempt suicide.[229] Substance abuse greatly complicates treatment[230] with a greater chance of hospitailisation,[231] a greater risk of lithium toxicity,[232] an increased chance of medication non-compliance[233] and an increased risk that meds will not work.[234]

All in all, alcohol and substance abuse/misuse definitely worsens the outcome for people with BP.[235]

Anxiety
What is anxiety?

Anxiety is the feeling we get when facing a perceived threat, like a job interview.[236] Anxiety is characterised by 'feelings of worry, nervousness, and unease',[237] it is anticipatory (future-focused), the result of expecting a stressful or painful upcoming possible event or situation.[238] Anxiety is the feeling of dread or foreboding you get when you think something bad is going to happen.

Anxiety is the most common mental health disorder in the world.[239]

What are anxiety disorders?

A certain amount of anxiety in daily life is normal, and even a healthy reaction to worrying stimulus, like the example of the job

---

[228] NCCMH, 2006:99.
[229] Marohn, 2011:6; Fieve, 2006:120; NCCMH, 2006:99.
[230] Suppes & Keck, 2005:7.22.
[231] Kennard, 2011:24.
[232] Suppes & Keck, 2005:7.22.
[233] Jónsdóttir et al., 2012.
[234] Kennard, 2011:24.
[235] Roberts et al., 2013:52; Marohn, 2011:6; McManamy, 2006:111.
[236] Roberts et al., 2013:135.
[237] Boyes, 2015:3.
[238] Roberts et al., 2013:133.
[239] Evans & Allen, 2009:183.

interview; though some people thrive in these types of stressful situation, most of us would be a little bit anxious.

Anxiety disorders on the other hand are not healthy, normal reactions to stimulus. They are a group of 'conditions marked by extreme or pathological anxiety or dread',[240] anxiety becomes an anxiety disorder when the level and frequency of anxiety becomes impairing and has an impact on day-to-day functioning.

Anxiety disorders can exist in isolation, but they are usually comorbid (co-existing) with other anxiety disorders or with affective disorders, like depression or bipolar.[241] Anxiety disorders are highly treatable, 'but only about one-third of sufferers receive treatment'.[242] Anxiety disorders may affect 18% of the population at any one time, and 30% will experience an anxiety problem over their lifetime.[243]

Some examples of anxiety disorders which co-occur with bipolar are: Generalised Anxiety Disorder (GAD), Social Phobia (Social Anxiety Disorder), Specific Phobia, Panic Disorder, Obsessive-Compulsive Disorder (OCD), and Post-Traumatic Stress Disorder (PTSD).[244]

What's the connection with BPII?

First of all, as already noted anxiety 'is a common feature of both [hypomania] and depression'.[245]

Secondly, anxiety disorders commonly co-occur with BPII.[246] According to various studies, between 31% and 81% of people with bipolar also experience anxiety or an anxiety disorder.[247]

---

[240] Evans & Allen, 2009:182.
[241] NICE, 2011:5.
[242] Evans & Allen, 2009:183.
[243] Roberts et al., 2013:133.
[244] NICE, 2011:5.
[245] Fast & Preston, 2012:28.
[246] Fletcher, 2017; Roberts et al., 2013:17; Fieve, 2006:163; Simon et al., 2004; Perugi et al., 1999.

Life With Bipolar Type Two

However, the 'precise nature of the relationship between anxiety and bipolar illness remains unclear'.[248] Regardless, anxiety is of significant 'clinical relevance' in the treatment of bipolar.[249]

How do you recognise anxiety? Symptoms and behaviours:

There are two main areas which help you to recognise whether you are experiencing anxiety: symptoms and behaviours. There are physical and emotional symptoms, and thoughts and overt behaviours.[250]

Some of the physical symptoms of anxiety are:[251]

- sweating
- exhaustion
- intensifying of the senses
- pounding heart
- nausea
- muscle tension
- headache
- shortness of breath
- dizziness
- tunnel vision
- goose bumps
- trouble sleeping
- dry mouth
- cold hands or feet
- jumpiness
- fatigue.

It is unlikely that you would experience all these symptoms at the same time; most people have an anxiety "finger print" where they

---

[247] Owen & Saunders, 2008:31; McManamy, 2006:104; Simon et al., 2004.
[248] Simon et al., 2004; Mondimore, 1999:118.
[249] Young et al., 1993.
[250] Boyes, 2015:5; Fast & Preston, 2012:28; Evans & Allen, 2009:182.
[251] Roberts et al., 2013:134-135; Miller, 2009:59; Owen & Saunders, 2008:31.

experience the same set of physical symptoms each time they get anxious. If you are experiencing a few of these symptoms at the same time, you are probably experiencing anxiety.

Some emotional symptoms of anxiety are:[252]

- a sense of worthlessness
- feelings of helplessness
- depression
- feeling stressed
- feelings of dread
- shame
- nervousness
- a sense of being detached from the situation
- feeling worried
- feeling apprehensive.

Again, it is unlikely that you will feel all these emotional symptoms at the same time, though these emotions tend to be more variable than the physical symptoms we experience during anxiety; they often depend on the situation. If you experience a few at the same time, it is relatively easy to recognise them as anxious emotions.

Examples of some anxious thought behaviours are:[253]

- fear of failure
- mentally replaying events, even before they've happened
- all-or-nothing thinking
- negative predictions
- blaming yourself inappropriately for things that have gone wrong
- imposing ultra-high standards on yourself.

---

[252] Boyes, 2015:5; Roberts et al., 2013:134; Evans & Allen, 2009:182; Miller, 2009:59.
[253] Boyes, 2015:multiple pages.

It is unlikely you will think in all these ways at the same time, but you may have recurrent thought patterns which you can use to identify when you're feeling anxious.

The most common overt anxious behaviour is avoidance, also known as prevention focus.[254] This is basically where you choose to not engage in situations that make you feel anxious or avoid the object of your anxiety. If you engage in avoidance it is likely you have anxiety.

Other anxious behaviours include:[255]

- procrastination
- hesitation
- paralysing perfectionism.

If you excessively procrastinate, hesitate to make decisions, or don't start tasks for fear of failure, you are probably experiencing anxiety.

Problems related to comorbid anxiety:

Comorbid anxiety with BP is often associated with a worse course of illness than for those without anxiety.[256] People with bipolar and anxiety are more likely to abuse alcohol, less responsive to lithium, have a younger age at onset of symptoms, spend less time euthymic (in stable mood), and most importantly are at higher risk of death by suicide.[257] If left untreated anxiety disorders can cause unnecessary suffering and severe functional impairment.[258]

Generalised Anxiety Disorder (GAD):

---

[254] Boyes, 2015:22; Roberts et al., 2013:137.
[255] Boyes, 2015:6.
[256] McManamy, 2006:104; Simon et al., 2004; Myers & Thase, 2000.
[257] Evans & Allen, 2009:183; McManamy, 2006:104; Simon et al., 2004; Young et al., 1993.
[258] Fieve, 2006:163; Simon et al., 2004.

GAD is a disorder where anxiety greatly exceeds normal levels. It is characterised by 'chronic, persistent, uncontrollable worry',[259] it is often overwhelming and 'out of proportion to the stimulus'[260] and is 'associated with heightened tension because of constant worry'.[261] Though GAD may be triggered by certain situations, such as travelling to a new location, GAD is also characterised by 'free-floating' anxiety[262] which arises with no apparent cause or trigger.

GAD can be mild and irritating or it can be 'severe and incapacitating'.[263] Either simply making some activities more challenging or flat out impossible.

Social Phobia (Social Anxiety Disorder):

Social Phobia is a chronic, marked dread, anxiety and/or self-consciousness in social and/or 'performance situations'.[264] Social Anxiety Disorder can "kick in" around strangers, or even become overwhelming around people the person knows well.[265]

Common situations that activate Social Phobia are public speaking, parties and using public toilets.

People who have Social Phobia are at significant risk of having another anxiety disorder or a mood disorder, such as depression or BP.[266]

Specific Phobia:

Specific Phobia is exactly what it sounds like; it is intense fear or anxiety about a specific thing or situation, such as arachnophobia (fear of spiders), agoraphobia (fear of open spaces), or

---

[259] Roberts et al., 2013:140.
[260] Evans & Allen, 2009:193.
[261] NICE, 2011:5.
[262] Fast & Preston, 2012:28; McManamy, 2006:105.
[263] Evans & Allen, 2009:193.
[264] Roberts et al., 2013:140; Evans & Allen, 2009:205.
[265] Evans & Allen, 2009:205.
[266] Evans & Allen, 2009:205; Perugi et al., 1999.

claustrophobia (fear of enclosed spaces).[267] In the case of Specific Phobia, the person will usually go out of their way to avoid the object or situation of their dread, to the point of interfering with daily life.

Panic Disorder:

There is a consistent relationship between panic and BPII,[268] in fact it is reckoned that '20.8% of [people] with bipolar disorder also [meet] the criteria for panic disorder'.[269]

Panic Disorder is essentially anxiety in its most severe form.[270] It is the condition where you have 'recurring, unforeseen panic attacks',[271] which cause 'intense apprehension and feelings of impending doom'.[272] A panic attack is a 'sudden surge of intense fear... accompanied by strong physical sensations'.[273] Generally, panic attacks peak at 10-20 minutes and rarely last longer than half an hour, though symptoms may persist for hours after.[274] Panic Disorder can have 'both chronic and remitting courses',[275] that is it can be constant or occasional.

Obsessive-Compulsive Disorder (OCD):

Some reports suggest a strong 'linkage between OCD and bipolar'.[276] People with OCD have a high chance of having other anxiety disorders, and mood disorders.[277]

People with OCD have 'frequent, intrusive, and troublesome thoughts and ideas' (obsessions)[278]. And they typically engage in

---

[267] Roberts et al., 2013:140; NICE, 2011:5.
[268] Himmelhoch, 1998.
[269] Myers & Thase, 2000.
[270] Evans & Allen, 2009:185.
[271] NICE, 2011:5.
[272] Evans & Allen, 2009:185.
[273] Roberts et al., 2013:141.
[274] Boyes, 2015:188; Evans & Allen, 2009:185.
[275] NICE, 2011:6.
[276] Myers & Thase, 2000.
[277] Perugi et al., 1999.
[278] Roberts et al., 2013:141; Evans & Allen, 2009:213.

'repetitive behaviours or mental acts' (compulsions) which may become ritualised, in an attempt to alleviate anxiety.[279]

'Obsessions and compulsions may be simple or complex and ritualised'.[280] Overt compulsive behaviours include checking, hand washing or switching lights on and off. Mental, or cognitive, acts may include counting, praying or mantras. Sometimes compulsions can become a major life activity, taking up hours of the day, impairing daily function and being particularly distressing.[281] Compulsions can also become dangerous: for example, excessive hand washing may cause dermatitis or a skin infection.

Post-Traumatic Stress Disorder (PTSD):

PTSD usually develops after a person witnesses or experiences a terrifying, life-threatening, or seriously traumatic event such as rape, murder, torture, a natural disaster, child abuse, domestic violence or war-time combat.[282]

A person with PTSD often experiences flash-backs, nightmares and a sense of reliving the event.[283] This anxiety disorder can have a significant effect on a person's daily functioning as they try to avoid any and all possible reminders of the event.

People with PTSD are 'at increased risk for developing other anxiety-, mood- and substance-related disorders – especially alcohol abuse'[284] and depression.

Overcoming anxiety:

The best way to start managing anxiety is self-help. I highly recommend 'The Anxiety Toolkit' (Boyes, 2015) and 'The Bipolar II Disorder Workbook' (Roberts et al., 2013). I have selected a few of

---

[279] Roberts et al., 2013:141; Evans & Allen, 2009:213.
[280] Evans & Allen, 2009:213.
[281] Evans & Allen, 2009:216.
[282] Roberts et al., 2013:141; Evans & Allen, 2009:197.
[283] Evans & Allen, 2009:197.
[284] Evans & Allen, 2009:198.

the techniques they suggest, as well as including some of my own and from other sources, but if you have anxiety problems, I suggest you read their books; they are incredibly helpful.

Some techniques:

- Learn time management skills, such as making to-do lists, 'setting realistic goals and grouping tasks into batches'.[285]
- Fake it till you make it! If you feel stressed or anxious, pretend you feel relaxed: lower your shoulders, breathe normally. You'll find faking it actually makes you feel calmer.[286]
- Start small, get bigger: Start off doing smaller/simpler anxiety provoking tasks, and then once you've done a couple of those, work your way up to bigger/more difficult tasks and situations.[287]
- Desensitisation: Also known as exposure therapy, this is where you expose yourself gradually to the thing or situation that makes you feel nervous. It is often best to do this with a mental health professional or 'trusted companion'.[288]
- Music: put on some music you like, and sing, dance, hum or just listen. Or even make some music yourself.[289]
- Body scan: sit or lie somewhere comfortable, close your eyes. Now starting from your toes try to become acutely aware of what you can feel; the pressure of your feet on the floor, the softness of your slippers and any other sensations. Then work your way up your body doing the same thing; feet, ankles, calves, knees etc.[290]
- Stretch and release: sit or lie somewhere comfortable. Then with each part of your body, starting with your feet,

---

[285] Evans & Allen, 2009:197.
[286] Boyes, 2015:134.
[287] Boyes, 2015:150-151.
[288] Evans & Allen, 2009:212-213.
[289] Miller, 2009:144.
[290] Roberts et al., 2013:148-149.

stretch out the muscles as far as you can for five seconds then release, wait five seconds in a relaxed state then move on to the next body part. When you get to your face stretch your mouth wide, raise your eyebrows, open your eyes as wide as possible. If you're in a public place, try doing it with just your toes and fingers, no one will notice.
- CBT self-help: CBT-based books for bipolar, depression and anxiety are all out there, go find them.[291] There are also a lot of online courses.

Anxiolytic medication:

Of course, if after some time (give it a couple of months of practice) you still find your anxiety is taking over your life, there are medications your doctor can prescribe. If you're seeing a psychiatrist it is best to go through them, if not, your GP may be willing to provide a prescription.

First of all, if you're not on an antidepressant they may offer you an SSRI or SNRI (more about antidepressants in Psychopharmacology').[292] Sometimes this calms symptoms of anxiety. The other class that may be offered are benzodiazepines[293] though in most cases these are only used in the short term to treat acute instances of anxiety[294] because they can be addictive. (More about benzodiazepines in 'Psychopharmacology'.)

Self-harm

Trigger warning: *this section is about a very delicate topic. If at any point you feel that you are being triggered towards compulsions to self harm, please stop reading. Either skip forward past 'Self harm' and 'Suicide' or go do something relaxing and enjoyable and make sure to have a nice hot drink. Do not come back to this section*

---

[291] NICE, 2011:17-18.
[292] NICE, 2011:18.
[293] Roberts et al., 2013:17; Evans & Allen, 2009:196; McManamy, 2006:251; Mondimore, 1999:118.
[294] NICE, 2011:18; Mondimore, 1999:118.

> *today. If you are experiencing a depressive or mixed episode and are prone to self harm you may wish to go to the harmless self harm part or skip this section altogether; that's fine: your safety should not be compromised by reading a book.*

If, however this section simply makes you feel uncomfortable, good. Self-harm is a difficult topic to think about if you've never experienced it yourself. If you have ever self-harmed and think you might again in the future, the harmless self-harm part is for you.

One topic which is barely even mentioned in almost every book and article I've ever read is self-harm and surprisingly it does not feature on the DSM's list of depressive symptoms. Personally, I think this is horrifically remiss, it beggars belief. Self-harm is a common symptom of multiple mental health disorders, including bipolar.[295] Self-harm is one of the most upsetting, most destructive and most dangerous of depressive symptoms, and also features strongly in mixed episodes. And self-harm is more common with bipolar disorder than most other psychiatric disorders.[296] One of the reasons it is so important to tackle self-harm is that people who self-harm have 'a 50- to 100-fold higher likelihood of dying by suicide in the 12-month period after an episode than people who do not self-harm'.[297]

What is self-harm?

Self-harm takes many forms and may or 'may not be related to suicide or attempted suicide'.[298] Some self-destructive behaviours such as reckless driving or binge eating can be viewed as self-harm,[299] if the intention is self-injury.[300] When people talk about self-harm we often think of self-mutilation by cutting, but there are several ways to self-harm. The following is a list of categories of self-

---

[295] NICE, 2013:6.
[296] NCCMH, 2006:93.
[297] NICE, 2013:6.
[298] NHS, 2016.
[299] Fast & Preston, 2012:30.
[300] NICE, 2013:6.

harm, as with all lists in this book it is not exhaustive and just to remind you, *if you are a self-harmer perhaps it's best to skip to the 'Harmless Self-harm' section.*

- Self-mutilation: usually this means lacerating (cutting) or scratching the skin, but also includes piercing oneself with needles, burning oneself with fire or cigarettes and other forms. If the intention is to feel pain, body modification such as piercing, tattoos and scarification can also be seen as self-mutilation. (If the intention is purely aesthetic/decorational, it is NOT self-harm, not everyone with their ears pierced is a self-harmer.)
- Abusing medications or drugs/self-poisoning: this is when someone deliberately takes too much (overdose) or not enough of their prescription meds, or abuses over the counter medicines by deliberately exceeding the recommended dosage. It can also apply to the (mis)use of street drugs.
- Alcohol abuse: drinking to excess (binge drinking) can be seen as self-harm.
- Extreme or risky behaviours: deliberately having unsafe sex, driving dangerously or engaging in street fights can be self-harm.

Why do people self-harm?

There are myriad reasons why people may self-harm, I profess to only knowing a few:

- As an outward expression of grief: some people use self-harm as a way of getting past the grief of a loss.
- To feel something: sometimes when people are depressed they go emotionally numb and can't feel. When this happens, we might seek physical sensations where we know the exact feeling and reaction we'll get from our bodies. We seek something tangible and real.

- For control: sometimes everyone feels like their whole world and life is completely out of their control and they have no power over anything. When someone with BPII feels like this, they may self-harm as a way of controlling something in their lives.[301]
- To punish ourselves: sometimes we use self-harm to punish ourselves for perceived wrongs we have committed; it is a form of self-flagellation.
- To distract ourselves: sometimes it is simply to distract ourselves from our psychological suffering.[302]

There may be several more reasons, but those are the ones I know exist.

What can you do instead of self-harm? /Harmless self-harm:

There are a lot of techniques called harmless self-harm. The idea is, when you feel the compulsion to self-harm you try at least one, preferably two or three, of these techniques to see if you can eradicate or reduce the urge to self-harm.

Some harmless self-harm techniques are:

- Putting tight rubber bands round your wrist and 'twanging' them against your skin.
- Working out until you physically hurt.
- Holding ice cubes in your hands until they completely melt.
- Using tweezers to pluck hair from sensitive body parts like armpits, groin and nose.
- Drawing hard lines on your skin in red pen.
- Drawing elaborate pictures or patterns on yourself using coloured pens (sharpies work particularly well).

---

[301] NHS, 2016.
[302] NHS, 2016; Fast & Preston, 2012:31.

- Dripping hot wax on your skin, somewhere like your thigh so it's easy to wipe away.

Or you can partake in a pleasurable sensual experience like having a bath or masturbating.

Or you can escape by going to bed and trying to sleep; when you feel like self-harming you are often emotionally exhausted, you may find it's easier to sleep than you think. You might not feel cheerful when you wake up, but you'll have been safe the whole time you were asleep.

Harmless self-harm techniques do not always work, but they're worth using every time you feel like self-harming, just in case it can prevent it that once. Perhaps each time you feel like self-harming you could try a different technique or get creative and come up with your own. Find what works for you.

What if it doesn't work?

The first thing to do if harmless self-harm techniques don't work on any particular occasion is set an alarm for 15 minutes time and go wash the dishes or sort paperwork or some other mundane activity. You may well find that by the time your alarm goes off the compulsions to self-harm have dissipated.

If that doesn't work, you are very likely to self-harm. So, try to limit yourself. I am not advocating self-harm to any degree, but if you have to self-harm put limits in place. For example, if you're going to cut yourself, just do one small shallow cut somewhere you're not likely to hit major blood vessels and then set another fifteen-minute alarm and go do another mundane thing. Again, you may well find one was enough and your compulsions have dissipated.

There are plenty of things you can try if you are worried you will self-harm, give them a go. I hope something works for you.

Suicide

*This section being dedicated to the topic of suicide, I am issuing another **trigger warning**:*

If you find the content of this section makes you feel compulsions or drives you to intention to commit suicide please stop reading and find yourself some company and something relaxing and distracting to do.

Depression, hypomania, mixed states and suicide:

Suicidal thoughts are a common symptom of both depression and mixed episodes.[303] A rapid switch from hypomania to depression is a time of particularly high risk.[304] It is not possible to rule out an impulsive suicide attempt taking place during a manic or hypomanic fit of irritability or by an act of over-confidence.[305]

What's the risk?

Suicide is a very real risk of having BPII,[306] 15% or more people with bipolar disorder die by suicide,[307] a ten to twenty times greater risk than the general population.[308] 24% to 50% of people with bipolar attempt suicide at least once,[309] with those with BPII at especially high risk.[310] 3% to 20% of those hospitalised for their bipolar symptoms go on to commit suicide. Annually around 0.4% of bipolar patients die by suicide.[311] It is worth emphasising that not all bipolar

---

[303] NHS, 2016; Kamba et al., 2011; Jackel, 2010; Evans & Allen, 2009:150; NCCMH, 2006:98; Yatham et al, 2005.

[304] NCCMH, 2006:93.

[305] Evans & Allen, 2009:153.

[306] NHS, 2016; Fast & Preston, 2012:30; Baek et al., 2011; Kennard, 2011:2; Haycock, 2010:xv & 103; Owen & Saunders, 2008:126; Fast, 2006; Suppes & Keck, 2005:4.19; Serretti et al., 2002.

[307] Haycock, 2010:xv; Owen & Saunders, 2008:126.

[308] NHS, 2016; Suppes & Keck, 2005:4.19.

[309] NHS, 2016; Haycock, 2010:103; Jackel, 2010; NCCMH, 2006:73.

[310] Baek et al., 2011; NCCMH, 2006:73; Serretti et al., 2002.

[311] NCCMH, 2006:73.

patients attempt to commit suicide[312] and this is significantly better than estimates as high as 60% from studies in the 1940s.[313]

It is easy to forget that bipolar disorder is a potentially lethal illness.[314] As such any suicide attempt or suicidal intention must be taken extremely seriously,[315] the person should be overseen in a safe environment[316] and a limited amount of medication should be prescribed to anyone who is suicidal.[317] The chapter 'Stability is the Goal' in this book is especially important for this reason, because 'relapse prevention is suicide prevention'.[318]

Why do people attempt suicide?

The two main reasons I have come across are guilt and self-hatred[319] or an attempt to end the suffering inflicted by bipolar episodes.[320] We sometimes feel guilty about becoming a "burden" to our families and friends, and society in general. We might feel guilty about any pain we have caused our loved ones. Or we may even feel guilty for being ill. But more often than not, suicide is simply seen as the only way to escape the pain and suffering.

What to do if you feel suicidal:

There are two categories of suicidal thoughts: passive and active.[321] Passive suicidal thoughts may simply be morbid thoughts like 'if I walked into the road I might get hit by a car', or 'I'd be better off dead'. Active suicidal thoughts are when you are making plans or taking actions towards your own death. The "protocol" is slightly

---

[312] Duke & Hochman, 1993:xxvi.
[313] Mondimore, 1999:238.
[314] Mondimore, 1999:232.
[315] Todd, 2016:15; Marohn, 2011:8; McManamy, 2006:190; Kessler et al., 2005; Mondimore, 1999:238.
[316] Evans & Allen, 2009:176.
[317] NCCMH, 2006:14.
[318] Mondimore, 1999:238.
[319] Fast & Preston, 2012:30.
[320] Fast & Preston, 2012:30; Marohn, 2011:173.
[321] Fast, 2006.

different depending in whether your suicidal thoughts are passive or active.

If your thoughts and feelings are passive it is best to not be alone.[322] Call a trusted friend or family member and explain that you are currently preoccupied with thoughts of death and suicide and need to not be alone. Explain that you are not in a good place and could really do with some company. If you are having passive suicidal ideation, then your loved ones (family/partner/close friends) should really know abut it. This way they can help to keep an eye on you and your symptoms in case your thoughts should become active and you need interventive care. It is also really important that your Care Co-ordinator (CPN or social worker), your psychiatrist and, If you have one, your psychologist/therapist know too, this way they can help to tailor your treatment and support.

If you are having active thoughts of suicide it is an emergency. Get yourself to A&E at your nearest hospital or go to the duty nurse at your mental health clinic.[323] Ideally get someone to go with you/take you there. If you go to A&E then you will most likely see a triage nurse, an A&E doctor, then the on-call psychiatrist or mental health team. If you go straight to your mental health clinic you will see the duty worker, then hopefully your own psychiatrist (if they're working that day); almost all mental health clinics keep a few appointments every week for emergency visits. Whoever you see will do an assessment and decide what kind of treatment or intervention you need; this might be an extra med for a few days, it might be management under the home treatment team for a while, or it might be going into a psychiatric unit for a short while. Whatever is decided, it is in your best interest, so don't be scared.

If you develop the intention to kill yourself you **must** tell someone as soon as possible and get yourself emergency help. Do not try to

---

[322] Fast, 2006.
[323] Miller, 2009:237.

> fight thoughts of suicide on your own. **Tell someone. Get help.** Suicide is a desperate last resort[324] and there is always help available somewhere with someone.

Sex & Hypersexuality

If you've read just about any other book about bipolar (I or II) they probably made two mentions about sex. First hyper-sexuality may have been listed as a symptom of mania or hypomania. Secondly, they mention sex when they discuss risky/damaging behaviours having a negative impact on relationships; specifically, infidelity. Two small mentions normally. I think sex is too important to have such a tiny place, so I've given it a section.

Hypomania:

A not uncommon symptom of the hypomanic state is hypersexuality, that is, a significantly increased sex drive or libido.[325] For some people who have partners who can keep up and enjoy a lot of sex, this may not be a problem. However, for a lot of people with BPII hypersexuality can become quite the issue. People with BPII have a higher risk of 'episodic promiscuity, extramarital affairs, or a compulsion toward sexual encounters'.[326] When hypomanic, sexual encounters and propositions 'may multiply',[327] and in many cases the notion of "safe sex" goes out the window, which can lead to unwanted pregnancies and sexually transmitted diseases.[328] Oftentimes, sexual advances may be made at inappropriate times or to inappropriate people due to the inhibition common in hypomania. Obviously, these risks are serious, but there are others. Bipolar driven hypersexuality can lead to destroyed relationships, loss of trust, lost jobs and/or broken homes.

---

[324] Moezzi, 2016.
[325] bpMagazine, 2016; Todd, 2016:22; Leader, 2013:14; Fast & Preston, 2012:173; Haycock, 2010:4; Fisher, 2008:114; Fieve, 2006:24; Duke & Hochman, 1993:161.
[326] Fieve, 2006:119.
[327] Leader, 2013:14.
[328] Fieve, 2006:116.

Of course, there are bonuses to hypersexuality: sex if often much more enjoyable, your senses are heightened, and the intensity can make sex 'sizzling'.[329] If your partner also enjoys a lot of sex, then hypersexuality can actually make your relationship stronger. Energetic sex is excellent exercise. And sex releases endorphins, the body's feel good chemicals, which can also help reduce feelings of pain.

Depression:

Oftentimes during depression, we go the opposite way and our sex drive (libido) decreases, which can become so severe that we shun all forms of physical intimacy. This can have just as damaging an effect on relationships as hypersexuality, causing harboured negative feelings and even generating guilt. Just try to remember that as the depression loses its grasp, your sex life will begin to return to normal. So, stick with any antidepressants you are prescribed and therapies you are referred to.

Some sex rules to live by:

Especially when you're in a mood state you need to be aware of your desires and try to stay safe when you are practising sex. Set yourself some rules and try to stick to them. Some good ones I've found are:

- Make sure you know the full name of anyone you intend to sleep with.
- Don't have sex if you're drunk.
- Always use barrier protection (condoms).
- If you take someone home, make sure to tell a friend and ask them to call you later to check you're ok.
- Get checked regularly for STIs and STDs.
- Always go to your place; it's safer.
- Don't have sex for self-punishment.

---

[329] bpMagazine, 2016; McManamy, 2006:91-98.

Please practise safe sexual practices even with long term partners, and keep yourself aware of what you're doing. But remember to have fun; if you're not enjoying it, stop it.

Catastrophising

Loads of people (with and without bipolar) catastrophise; but in my experience, and from talking to other people with BPII, we do it all the time and it leads to such terrible anxiety. Catastrophising is basically when we "make a mountain out of a molehill"; in our minds we make everything lead to the most terrible outcome that it could, often completely by accident.

There are really two groups of catastrophising; I call them Type A and Type B, "logical" and "illogical" catastrophising.

Type A: Logical catastrophising...

Sometimes my catastrophising (and a lot of people's) takes perfectly logical but wildly exaggerated steps.

E.g. I don't get to sleep until midnight and I'm wide awake at three in the morning because my knees are causing me a lot of pain. Cue catastrophising:

1. I won't be able to get back to sleep because I'm in pain.
2. I'll be sore and tired in the morning.
3. I won't have the energy or physical ability to get down the stairs.
4. I won't have breakfast so I'll be hungry.
5. I'll have even less energy.
6. I won't leave the house, so I won't go to CBT.
7. I'll miss CBT.
8. They will think I don't take CBT seriously.
9. I'll be discharged.
10. I won't have that support structure.
11. I'll get worse again.
12. I won't be able to leave the house, so I'll get isolated again.
13. I'll get lonely and restless.

14. I'll get sad.
15. I'll get suicidal.
16. So I'll kill myself.

See I went from being sore and awake really early to believing this meant I would kill myself soon. The steps are logical, but so exaggerated as to be unrealistic. I mean, it could happen, but it is **so** unlikely.

Type B: Illogical catastrophising...

Type B is much more difficult to follow. There are steps but some of them don't make sense to a healthy mind; to most people the train of thought just wouldn't make sense.

E.g. I forget to put a load of laundry in the machine before I go out. Cue catastrophising:

1. I won't have anything to wear tomorrow that's clean {not true, I would have a wardrobe full of clean clothes}.
2. I will smell bad and my partner will notice.
3. He will hate it and never want to see me again.
4. All my friends will hear about how bad I smell.
5. I will be alone forever.
6. My parents will kick me out for being unhygienic.
7. I'll be homeless and alone.
8. I won't be able to get my medications.
9. I'll get really ill and no one will notice or care.
10. I'll die on the streets with no one knowing who I am or where I come from.

So... If I forget to put a load of laundry in the machine, realistically either I put it in when I get home or my folks are likely to put it in. If not I do have plenty of clothes, the likelihood of me having absolutely nothing clean is slim. But bipolar brain did this to me once. I managed to get from not putting in one load of laundry to being a dead, nameless, homeless person. Logically, this series of events is never going to happen, but on that day my brain worked against me. I ended up getting off the bus, turning round and going home to put on the laundry which made me late for meeting a friend so I just cancelled instead. So my catastrophising actually led to a negative outcome which had nothing to do with the problematic train of thought. Ironic really.

But as you can see, catastrophising is just massively unhelpful and unhealthy. At best, you end up a little nervous and play that train of thought around and around in your head. At worst, you cause something bad to happen by trying to protect yourself from something else. I know a woman who tried to break off her engagement because she had a "fat day" and convinced herself that her fiancé was cheating on her because she was ugly. (Thankfully he had none of it.)

Nothing good comes out of catastrophising.

Fixing your catastrophising

The only way I've found to bring myself back from catastrophising is to challenge each step. I try to notice if any of the steps in my train of thought don't make much sense and challenge the idea with a more logical reaction or step. If I can't do it for that step, I try for the next one, and so on. It can work, it might not. When it does, that's great, obviously. When it doesn't, I end up having an anxious day and avoiding anything connected to that unhelpful train of thought. In which case I use my techniques for overcoming anxiety.

Chapter Three:

Treatment

Without Treatment

Bipolar disorder type two, as I said and has been confirmed by researchers and psychiatrists around the globe, is manageable. However, it being so difficult to diagnose and people waiting up to a decade for diagnosis, means many more people are left untreated, undertreated or mis-treated for a long time.

Undiagnosed and/or untreated BPII can wreak havoc on lives;[330] it can cause problems at work, at school and in the home; it can destroy relationships, result in prison, hospitalisation, bankruptcy, and even death (either by suicide or tragic accident).[331]

People 'do not develop a tolerance to [mood disorders] or become more resilient over time. On the contrary, the evidence points to increased sensitivity to events or situations that trigger relapse'.[332] The bulk of evidence suggests that if left untreated, the course of bipolar disorder worsens over time with symptoms becoming more severe and episodes more frequent.[333] And furthermore, the more mood episodes you have, 'the more difficult the disorder is to treat' over time.[334]

So the moral of the story is: if you think you or a loved one has bipolar disorder (BPI or BPII), get an appointment with the GP, go armed with your list of symptoms and any previous meds or diagnoses you've had, and ask to be referred to psychiatric services. A good GP will oblige.

Psychiatrists

If you go to your GP and they think you may have BPII (or any other psychiatric disorder for that matter) then they should refer you to

---

[330] Nichols, 2016.
[331] bipolarUK, 2018; APA, 2017; Fletcher, 2017; NHS, 2016; Haycock, 2010:2 & 251; Evans & Allen, 2009:152; Miklowitz et al., 2007b.
[332] Kennard, 2011:20.
[333] Mehta, 2016; Marohn, 2011:5.
[334] Roberts et al., 2013:112.

Mental Health Services (MHS) for an assessment with a psychiatrist.[335] From that point on a psychiatrist should supervise your psychiatric (mental health) treatment.[336] In particular psychiatrists manage medication and make referrals for psychotherapy and other interventions.[337]

The first part of a psychiatrist's role is the assessment and diagnosis of a patient brought into MHS. It is notoriously difficult to diagnose BPII; the clinician must know about a very specific set of signs and symptoms,[338] which means they must conduct a thorough assessment. When 'assessing suspected bipolar disorder healthcare professionals should:

- take a full history including family history, a review of all previous episodes and any symptoms between episodes
- assess the patient's symptom profile, triggers to previous episodes, social and personal functioning, comorbidities including substance misuse and anxiety, risk, physical health, and current psychosocial stressors
- obtain where possible, and within the bounds of confidentiality, a corroborative history from a family member or carer
- consider using formal criteria including self-rating scales such as the Mood Disorder Questionnaire.'[339]

Right from the beginning of the care relationship between patient and psychiatrist, the psychiatrist should 'build supportive and empathic relationships as an essential part of care'.[340] It is really important that you and your psychiatrist develop a collaborative relationship where you are actively involved in the decision-making

---

[335] NICE, 2014:16; NCCMH, 2006:12.
[336] Railton, 2016; Hodges, 2012:50.
[337] APA, 2017; Hodges, 2012:50.
[338] Fieve, 2006:162.
[339] NCCMH, 2006:13.
[340] NICE, 2014:13; NCCMH, 2006:10-11.

process at every stage of your treatment right from diagnosis.[341]

The second stage of a psychiatrist's role is to stabilise the acute episode (your initial presenting mood state). Usually this takes the form of medication; for example, for a major depression this may be a mood stabiliser combined with an antidepressant (more about medication coming up).

Once the initial mood episode is generally under control and symptoms have alleviated somewhat, the next part of a psychiatrist's role is the development of both maintenance and crisis plans, with the assistance and decision-making capacity of the person with BPII fully taken into account. A risk management plan (maintenance and crisis plan combined) should include:

- 'identifying personal, social, occupational or environmental triggers and early warning signs and symptoms of relapse
- a protocol for applying the person's own coping strategies and increasing doses of medication or taking additional medication (which can be given to the person in advance) for people at risk of onset of mania or for whom early warning signs and symptoms can be identified
- agreement between primary and secondary care about how to respond to an increase in risk or concern about possible risk
- information about who to contact if the person with bipolar disorder and, if appropriate, their carer, is concerned or in crisis, including the names of healthcare professionals in primary and secondary care who can be contacted.

Give the person and their GP a copy of the plan, and encourage the person to share it with their carers.'[342]

---

[341] NHS, 2016; NICE, 2014:7; NCCMH, 2006:16.
[342] NICE, 2014:20-21.

Maintenance treatment (long term treatment) arranged and supervised by your psychiatrist may include: a medications regimen, referrals to psychotherapy services and engagement with the Community Mental Health Team (CMHT) through Community Psychiatric Nurses (CPNs), social workers, and regular outpatient appointments. As well as managing your medications, your psychiatrist makes referrals for psychological interventions, such as CBT, and engaging the involvement of CMHT in maintenance care in the community.

15:9

Personally, I've seen 15 psychiatrists in nine years. The longest time I've ever kept the same psychiatrist is two years; most I've only seen once or twice. The reason for this: locums. A locum doctor is the same concept as a supply teacher; they cover periods of sickness and temporarily fill positions that can't be filled with permanent staff. Nowadays, psychiatry on the NHS seems to rely on locums. Most clinics seem to have one permanent clinician and then a series of locums filling the other posts. For this reason, it is not at all unusual to see two or three psychiatrists over the course of a single year. As you can imagine, this causes some difficulties. There is no "continuity of care", which first and most importantly means your psychiatrists never get to know you, and you never get to know them. This makes it difficult for you to build any real trust and means they don't develop a bank of knowledge about you and your bipolar. The other main problem comes from the fact that each psychiatrist is an individual just as much as we are individuals as patients; this means that they may have their own preferences toward treatment structures, they may like certain meds over others and may have different approaches to problems. So, often, each time you see a locum, they want to change something put in place by the last locum.

Good doctors, bad doctors & tablets doctors

To my mind there are three categories of psychiatrist; good, bad and tablets doctors. Never have I met a simply satisfactory psychiatrist.

Good doctors:

Good psychiatrists I believe can be recognised within minutes of first meeting them. They start each appointment by actually greeting you and asking how you are. I think most of us would recognise this as a good start.

Then, if it's your first appointment with MHS, their assessment procedure actually covers all the content above and they take notes as they go. They also ask probing, sensible questions like 'Why do you want this appointment?', 'In your opinion, what doesn't seem right?' and 'What would you like to come out of this appointment?'; all good open-ended questions which give you the opportunity to say your piece, and where even the answer 'I'm not sure' is helpful to the clinician. You get to contribute to the conversation; a good psychiatrist tries to have a proper two-way conversation.

If you're not new to MHS, but it's the first time you're seeing this doctor, they will have read your notes and will only ask you a few corroborating questions rather than conducting a whole new initial assessment for their own benefit.

By the time you've seen a good psychiatrist twice they have built a good rapport with you, you feel not only like you can trust them, but also that they trust and respect you, and they are treating you, rightly so, as the leading authority on your illness.

Right from the very first time you meet them, a good psychiatrist includes you in the decision-making process; they don't just make decisions and expect you to agree like a lost lamb. A good doctor makes recommendations, explaining why, and always tries to give you options.

NCCMH (National Collaborating Centre for Mental Health) recommendations state: 'Healthcare professionals should aim to develop a therapeutic relationship with all patients with bipolar disorder, and advise them on careful and regular self-monitoring of symptoms (including triggers and early warning signs), lifestyle (including sleep hygiene and work patterns) and coping strategies.'[343]

NICE guidance states that good care should include: -working to develop a collaborative relationship; -providing written information; -encouraging self-help and support group attendance; -advising patients about recognising symptoms; -writing Advanced Directives (more later); -taking into account the needs of family and carers.[344] A good doctor will follow these guidelines.

Bad doctors:

Bad psychiatrists are just as easy to spot. They are rude and abrupt; they don't greet you warmly and they don't ask how you are so much as what's "wrong" with you.

If it's your first appointment with MHS, they do an initial assessment, but don't cover everything described above and it feels rushed.

If it's your first appointment with them, even if you've been seen by MHS before, they will insist on doing another poorly conducted initial assessment, which again, feels rushed.

A bad psychiatrist only asks closed questions (questions with only yes/no answers). And if you ever say 'I don't know', you are met with a huff or an exasperated sigh as though you are deliberately making their job more difficult.

---

[343] NCCMH, 2006:11.
[344] NHS, 2016.

There is no empathy or understanding from a bad doctor, instead you feel judged and patronised. They treat you like a clueless child. A bad psychiatrist does not ask for your opinion on treatment options, simply tells you what is going to happen and doesn't explain why. They do not respect you or trust your judgement.

I have unfortunately met my fair share of bad doctors in nine years; I'd say about a third of them.

What can you do if you do get a bad doctor? Well first you can try talking to them about how you feel. Say something like, 'Last session you made me feel uncomfortable and patronised because you weren't asking for my opinion or using my own knowledge of my illness'. They may change their attitude. If that doesn't work or is too daunting, you could try talking to your Care Co-ordinator or GP who can talk with the psychiatrist on your behalf. If neither of these work or appeal to you, the other option is to ask to see another psychiatrist. The way you do this is by speaking to the medical secretary (usually also the receptionist) or to the clinic manager at your psychiatrist's office. You do not have to give a reason why, but feedback is always helpful for other patients in the long-run.

Tablets doctors:

The third group are the tablets doctors. These are often more difficult to spot initially as they can ostensibly be good doctors or bad doctors. It is not their ability to assess, communicate or involve you in conversation that brings them under my fire, it is their approach to treatment. There are fewer of them around now, but if you get assigned a tablets doctor, prepare to become a guinea pig.

Tablets psychiatrists are stuck a couple of decades behind modern psychiatry: they ignore the role of psychotherapy in the treatment of bipolar and focus purely on meds.

This can go one of two ways: One, they can be "stickers", as in they put you on a meds regimen (often without asking your opinion of it) and force you to stick to it no matter what. They can ignore side effects and efficacy (or inefficacy) because it's one of their preferred drugs and they want to see how it pans out, no matter what it's like for you. Two, they are "tweakers", as in they are constantly adding, removing and changing the doses and timings of medications. Again ignoring what works or doesn't work for you and simply recording the side effects, but doing nothing about them. They just keep changing things.

Both stickers and tweakers rely solely on medication, but it's more like they're conducting research than treating a live human being.

Have a little faith

Most of the time these days I hope psychiatrists are good doctors, but regrettably bad doctors still exist. That being said, don't go into an appointment assuming you'll get a bad or a tablets doctor, keep an open mind. Doctors go through a lot of training to become psychiatrists: after 5 years of General Medical Training, they then take a 2-year Graduate Foundation Course, then they spend 6 years in psychiatric training.[345] So try to trust your psychiatrist if you can,[346] they really should know what they're doing.

Psychopharmacology (psychiatric medication)

In modern medicine the first step in the treatment of bipolar disorder is usually medication[347] particularly since most of the time treatment tends to commence during an acute, severe mood episode so symptoms need to be gotten under control quickly. If a person is diagnosed as BPII whilst experiencing mild or no mood symptoms then they may make the decision with their psychiatrist

---

[345] Owen & Saunders, 2008:108.
[346] Paquette, 2016.
[347] White, 2014:11; Owen & Saunders, 2008:57.

to not start meds, but instead to be closely monitored for a few months,[348] but this is unusual.

Medication is not only used to treat the acute phases of BPII, but usually once the presenting mood episode is under some control, a course of maintenance treatment (long term treatment) will be put into action.[349] Usually meds are not the only treatment during the maintenance phase; typically a long term treatment plan also includes psychotherapy as this too has been shown to improve outcomes.[350]

Many people with bipolar view their medications as essential to their well-being and stability,[351] but whether or not to take meds is a personal choice,[352] though it is not a decision to take lightly and should be made with your psychiatrist.

Trial and error

Mental 'illness is not an exact science',[353] it is often the case that a psychiatrist must use their best judgement based on the available information about each patient as each person is an individual with their own history of episodes and symptoms and their own unique biochemistry.[354] There 'is an art to ... finding the precise medications to stabilize each patient, while allowing them to continue functioning at the highest possible level'.[355] As such, it takes time, effort and a degree of good luck to find the right treatment(s) for each person with BPII.[356] Usually finding the right

---

[348] Fieve, 2006:160.
[349] Todd, 2016:46; Fast & Preston, 2012:52; Bauer et al., 2006; NCCMH, 2006:281.
[350] Roberts et al., 2013:20; Bauer et al., 2006; NCCMH, 2006:281.
[351] Todd, 2016:46.
[352] Chellingsworth & Farrand, 2015:50.
[353] White, 2014:13.
[354] Haycock, 2010:73; Guyol, 2006:214.
[355] Fieve, 2006:27.
[356] Owen & Saunders, 2008:58.

medication regimen takes a lot of trial and error[357] and requires a great deal of patience.[358] Most people with bipolar will try more than one med to find the right one for them.[359] More than 50% of antidepressant users try more than two meds, and 10% try five or more,[360] and that is to say nothing of the other meds used to treat bipolar. It can take quite a long time, in some rare cases over a decade, to find the right meds combination (cocktail).[361] In fact, it is so common that people either don't tolerate or receive no benefit from their first medication(s) that the NICE guidelines even point out to psychiatrists that they may need to offer an alternative antipsychotic after a failed first prescription.[362]

What meds are used to treat BPII?

The four main groups of medications used to treat BPII are: mood stabilisers, antipsychotics, antidepressants and anxiolytics (anti-anxiety meds).[363]

Mood stabilisers:

The three main mood stabilisers used to treat BPII are: lithium,[364] valproate[365] and lamotrigine.[366] Mood stabilisers aim to smooth out mood episodes and reduce recurrences.[367]

Lithium

---

[357] APA, 2017; White, 2014:12; Roberts et al., 2013:15; Hall-Flavin, 2012; Guyol, 2006:14.
[358] Todd, 2016:47.
[359] Fast & Preston, 2012:30; Haycock, 2010:109.
[360] McManamy, 2006:218.
[361] Paquette, 2016; Fast & Preston, 2012:37.
[362] NICE, 2014:72.
[363] APA, 2017; Railton, 2016; White, 2014:11-12; Fast & Preston, 2012:36; Hall-Flavin, 2012; Hodges, 2012:71; Kennard, 2011:19; Owen & Saunders, 2008:57; Fieve, 2006:189; Suppes & Keck, 2005:8.2.
[364] Railton, 2016; Hodges, 2012:71; Kennard, 2011:19; Fieve, 2006:187.
[365] Railton, 2016; Hodges, 2012:71; Kennard, 2011:19; Suppes & Keck, 2005:8.2.
[366] Railton, 2016; Hodges, 2012:71; Kennard, 2011:19.
[367] Nichols, 2016; Fieve, 2006:188-189.

Lithium is the most commonly prescribed medication used to treat bipolar disorder.[368] It is the only "true" mood stabiliser in that it wasn't first developed as an anticonvulsant.[369] Lithium is still regarded as the most reliable mood stabiliser[370] as it is a very effective medication for a lot of people.[371] Some estimates put the efficacy of lithium as high as 60% to 80%[372] and it is thus considered the first line of treatment for most people with bipolar.[373]

Lithium has been shown to be particularly effective against treating mania and hypomania, but less so against acute episodes of bipolar depression.[374] Though it does have an excellent track record for the prevention of all bipolar mood episodes.[375]

One reason lithium is so popular as a maintenance medication for BP is that it is non-addictive.[376] Though effectiveness onset usually takes around two weeks, longer than the anticonvulsants used as mood stabilisers.[377] So, many psychiatrists prescribe a short course of another mood stabiliser at a high dose to help things settle down whilst waiting for the lithium to come into effect.

Lithium is not, however, considered especially good for treating mixed episodes or rapid cycling, though it is often on par with the other available mood stabilisers – the anticonvulsants.[378]

Lithium has an excellent reputation for reducing the number of suicides and suicide attempts compared with those not receiving

---

[368] NHS, 2016.
[369] Roberts et al., 2013:16; McManamy, 2006:229.
[370] Kennard, 2011:22.
[371] Hodges, 2012:71.
[372] Kennard, 2011:34; Duke & Hochman, 1993:141.
[373] NICE, 2014:27.
[374] Evans & Allen, 2009:158; Mondimore, 1999:87.
[375] Fast & Preston, 2012:219.
[376] Fast & Preston, 2012:221.
[377] NCCMH, 2006:205; Duke & Hochman, 1993:144.
[378] Ghaemi, 2008.

Life With Bipolar Type Two

treatment.[379]

No one knows exactly why lithium works as a mood stabiliser, but the important fact is that it does.[380]

It is important when you are on lithium to avoid taking non-steroidal anti-inflammatories like ibuprofen or diclofenac.[381]

History of Lithium:

After a fashion, lithium's heling effects were discovered at least 2,000 years ago by Ancient Greek and Roman physicians. They used to send people to hot springs for any number of physical and psychological ailments. Many of these springs were lithium-rich waters.[382]

Coming forward to modern medicine, John Cade in Australia accidentally stumbled across lithium's anti-manic effects when using it as a carrying agent for other chemicals and compositions.[383]

In 1954, Mogens Schou in Denmark conducted the first lithium double-blind study and became convinced that lithium could not only treat evident episodes of bipolar, but could prevent new episodes from occurring as well.[384] In 1967 he performed another trial which confirmed his hypothesis.[385]

By 1970 the usefulness of this 'simple element had been established',[386] so it was granted FDA approval in America.[387]

---

[379] NCCMH, 2006:248
[380] Suppes & Keck, 2005:8.3; Duke & Hochman, 1993;144.
[381] NHS, 2016.
[382] Mondimore, 1999:84.
[383] Haycock, 2010:31; Suppes & Keck, 2005:8.3; Duke & Hochman, 1993: 141.
[384] Mondimore, 1999:85; Duke & Hochman, 1993:141.
[385] Mondimore, 1999:85.
[386] Haycck, 2010:31.
[387] Roberts et al., 2013:16; Suppes & Keck, 2005:8.3; Duke & Hochman, 1993:143.

Monitoring:

If the lithium levels in your blood stream get too high there is a risk of you developing toxicity which can cause irreparable damage to your organs. Because of this it is vitally important that anyone on lithium has regular blood tests to check their levels.[388] Another reason to have regular blood tests is to check your kidney and thyroid functions.[389]

Side effects:

Arguably the most significant risk factor of lithium treatment is the long term possibility of developing renal (kidney) failure,[390] this is why it is so important to keep up-to-date with your blood tests.

However, the most common side effects reported by those on lithium are mental slowing and impaired concentration,[391] but most of the time these side effects can be reduced or even eliminated with proper management of the dose quantity and timing.[392]

A common concern is that lithium will dull the senses and impair creativity; in fact, a 1970 review of artists on lithium revealed that 75% claimed lithium treatment 'did not affect, or else improved, their creativity'.[393]

Lithium is a diuretic and can cause constipation; as such it is important to eat plenty of fibre,[394] and stay well hydrated.[395]

Valproate

---

[388] Wooldridge, 2016:30; McManamy, 2006:229; Suppes & Keck, 2005:8.10-8.11.
[389] NHS, 2016; Roberts et al., 2013:16; Hodges, 2012:72.
[390] McManamy, 2006:229.
[391] Jamison, 1993:243.
[392] McManamy, 2006:230; Mondimore, 1999:90.
[393] Haycock, 2010:52.
[394] White, 2014:67.
[395] McManamy, 2006:229.

Valproate, or valproic acid, is an anticonvulsant used as a mood stabiliser for people with bipolar.[396] Valproate is particularly used for bipolar manic episodes[397] and is reportedly better than lithium and some other meds for the treatment of bipolar mixed episodes.[398] Valproate does not appear to have strong antidepressant effects.[399] Some comparison trials have demonstrated that valproate has 'antipsychotic as well as antimanic activity'.[400] Valproate is particularly prescribed for those who cannot take or do not tolerate lithium.[401]

Valproate's side effect profile is milder than lithium's,[402] but the list is still quite long: it is a notorious weight gainer,[403] has a risk of toxicity so requires regular blood tests[404] and carries the severe risk of causing birth defects such as spina bifida, heart abnormalities and cleft lip,[405] so if you are a woman of child-bearing age a frank conversation about your desires or chances for pregnancy must be had. Valproate can also interact poorly with a number of other meds, chiefly Aspirin, Wellbutrin and Lamotrigine, so do be careful to ensure that your psychiatrist has a list of all the medications you are on before you start taking Valproate. And don't miss your regular blood tests.

Lamotrigine

Lamotrigine is an anticonvulsant (anti-epileptic drug) which acts as a mood stabiliser for those with BP.[406] It is one of several

---

[396] Haycock, 2010:71.

[397] Mondimore, 1999:93.

[398] McManamy, 2006:230; Suppes & Keck, 2005:8.12; Mondimore, 1999:94.

[399] McManamy, 2006:230; Suppes & Keck, 2005:9.6; Mondimore, 1999:94.

[400] Suppes & Keck, 2005:8.12.

[401] Evans & Allen, 2009:158; Owen & Saunders, 2008:76.

[402] Mondimore, 1999:94.

[403] McManamy, 2006:231.

[404] NHS, 2016; McManamy, 2006:231.

[405] NHS, 2016; NCCMH, 2006:207.

[406] Haycock, 2010:72.

anticonvulsants used to help manage BPII.

Lamotrigine is often hailed as the best mood stabiliser for tackling bipolar depression.[407] Lamotrigine is also particularly good for alleviating mixed episodes and rapid cycling.[408]

Lamotrigine is often prescribed for BPII alone[409] or in combination with lithium or an antipsychotic.[410] A number of studies 'indicate that lamotrigine works well with other mood stabilizers in treatment-resistant patients'.[411]

Lamotrigine has a very favourable side effect profile, especially with a low incidence of weight gain.[412] Very importantly however, if you begin to develop a skin rash whilst taking lamotrigine see your GP immediately.[413] In very rare cases taking lamotrigine can result in the development of Stevens-Johnson syndrome[414] which is marked by a severe skin rash. Again, it is rare, but it is very serious; so if you begin taking lamotrigine and develop any form of rash, go see your GP. It's better to be safe than sorry.

Antipsychotics:

The three main antipsychotics now used to treat BPII are: olanzapine, quetiapine and risperidone. Despite what the name implies, these meds are not only used to curb psychotic symptoms, but also have mood stabilising properties.

Olanzapine

---

[407] Fast & Preston, 2012:222; Owen & Saunders, 2008:76; Fieve, 2006:189-190; McManamy, 2006:232; NCCMH, 2006:25; Suppes & Keck, 2005:9.4; Mondimore, 1999:97.
[408] Haycock, 2010:72; Fieve, 2006:189.
[409] NCCMH, 2006:26.
[410] Roberts et al., 2013:16; NCCMH, 2006:9.
[411] Mondimore, 1999:98.
[412] McManamy, 2006:233; Mondimore, 1999:98.
[413] NHS, 2016.
[414] McManamy, 2006:233; Suppes & Keck, 2005:9.5.

Olanzapine was the first atypical antipsychotic to receive American FDA and NHS approval for the treatment of bipolar and is the one which has been most studied in terms of its effect on mania.[415] It is part of the family of drugs know as atypical antipsychotics, or new generation antipsychotics,[416] called these names to differentiate them from the older antipsychotics of the 1950s and '60s.[417]

Usually taken for long term/maintenance treatment for BP it is in tablet form, however it can also be used by injection to calm intense agitation during an acute mixed or manic episode.[418] It is particularly effective for first line treatment when 'symptoms are severe and behaviour is disturbed'.[419]

In addition to olanzapine's antimanic effects, some studies have shown a 'modest but significant antidepressive effect'.[420]

As with many meds for bipolar, olanzapine is known to cause weight gain[421] and it is not recommended that you have any grapefruit as it may interfere with the effects of the med.[422]

Quetiapine

Quetiapine is another of the atypical antipsychotics[423] classified separately from the typical antipsychotics of the mid-twentieth century.[424]

It has a much better side effect profile than the older generation antipsychotics, though weight gain is an issue.

---

[415] Owen & Saunders, 2008:79; NCCMH, 2006:206; Suppes & Keck, 2005:8.27.
[416] Mondimore, 1999:114.
[417] Roberts et al., 2013:16.
[418] Haycock, 2010:76.
[419] NHS, 2016; Owen & Saunders, 2008:79; NCCMH, 2006:9.
[420] McManamy, 2006:238.
[421] Haycock, 2010:76; NCCMH, 2006:206.
[422] Fast & Preston, 2012:227.
[423] Mondimore, 1999:114.
[424] Roberts et al., 2013:16.

In America and the UK quetiapine is licensed and approved for use with bipolar disorder, especially as an antimanic drug[425] because of its success in alleviating symptoms of mania.[426] It has also been found to have antidepressant effects.[427] Quetiapine is not just used for acute illness but also for maintenance treatment.

As with other atypical antipsychotics, grapefruit should be avoided.[428]

Risperidone

Risperidone is one of the atypical antipsychotics used to help manage BPII.

In 2003 the American FDA approved risperidone for use in treating acute mania and mixed episodes,[429] and in the UK for acute mania.[430] It is particularly indicated for these purposes[431] and can be safely combined with a number of antidepressants. And it also reduces cycle acceleration.[432]

The side effect profile is pretty good[433] though weight gain is often an issue.[434] It is best however, to avoid grapefruit and its derivatives as they 'may interfere with the effects' of the medication.[435]

Antidepressants:

Antidepressants (ADs) are a collection of medications which

---

[425] Roberts et al., 2013:17; McManamy, 2006:239; NCCMH, 2006:206.
[426] Haycock, 2010:76; Owen & Saunders, 2008:79.
[427] NHS, 2016; McManamy, 2006:239; NCCMH, 2006:245.
[428] Fast & Preston, 2012:227.
[429] McManamy, 2006:239.
[430] NCCMH, 2006:206.
[431] NHS, 2016; Haycock, 2010:76; Owen & Saunders, 2008:79; Suppes & Keck, 2005:8.29.
[432] Owen & Saunders, 2008:79.
[433] Owen & Saunders, 2008:79; Suppes & Keck, 2005:8.29.
[434] Haycock, 2010:76.
[435] Fast & Preston, 2012:227.

alleviate or reduce depressive symptoms. Usually these drugs impact the brain's neurotransmitter function in some way, causing a reduction in depression and a rise in mood.

There are three main types of antidepressants used to treat BPII: Selective-Serotonin Reuptake Inhibitors (SSRIs), Monoamine Oxidase Inhibitors (MAOIs), and Tricyclic Antidepressants (TCAs). Also slowly increasingly being used are Selective-Noradrenalin Reuptake Inhibitors (SNRIs).

ADs usually take a few weeks to fully get into the system and become properly effective.[436]

ADs in BPII

Antidepressants are sometimes used to treat bipolar depression.[437] Though technically no ADs are licensed in the UK for use in the treatment of BPII, so this is what's called "off-label use"[438] and is perfectly legal. Usually antidepressants are prescribed alongside a mood stabiliser to reduce the risk of "switching" (discussed below).[439]

The generally accepted wisdom is that after an acute episode of bipolar depression has been treated 'patients should not routinely continue on antidepressant treatment long-term';[440] however, because people with BPII 'are more prone to depression than hypomania' it is common for us to be treated long term with an antidepressant along with a mood stabiliser.[441]

All that being said, the role of ADs is still controversial.[442] Some

---

[436] Chellingsworth & Farrand, 2015:49.
[437] Evans & Allen, 2009:159; McManamy, 2006:246; Mondimore, 1999:100.
[438] NCCMH, 2006:250.
[439] Roberts et al., 2013:16; McManamy, 2006:246.
[440] NCCMH, 2006:10.
[441] Roberts et al., 2013:16.
[442] NCCMH, 2006:199-200.

think that antidepressants' risks do not outweigh the benefits,[443] where others feel that the benefits outweigh the risks.[444] '[These] opposing arguments centre on five issues': the risk of antidepressant-induced switching; the risk of antidepressant-induced cycle acceleration; the effectiveness of ADs in acute depression; the effectiveness of ADs in the prevention of relapse; and whether ADs actually reduce the risk of suicide in bipolar disorder.[445]

One thing that is agreed is that if a person becomes manic or hypomanic whilst taking an antidepressant, the antidepressant should be stopped.[446] And ADs should be avoided if a person is rapid cycling or has recently had a hypo episode.[447] It is also worth noting that if you are taking an antidepressant you should avoid 5-HTP, cimitedine, St John's wort and MAOIs (if taking another class of AD).[448]

SSRIs

Selective-Serotonin Reuptake Inhibitors, or SSRIs, are the most commonly prescribed ADs currently on the market. They do very much what it says on the tin; they work on the neurotransmitter serotonin. They block the reuptake of serotonin by the brain,[449] that is they reduce the amount which is reabsorbed by the brain increasing the concentration 'near its site of action in the brain'.[450]

SSRIs are commonly prescribed for both unipolar and bipolar depression and usually have a positive effect on both.[451] SSRIs have

---

[443] McManamy, 2006:245; NCCMH, 2006:245.
[444] McManamy, 2006:246; NCCMH, 2006:245.
[445] NCCMH, 2006:245-248.
[446] NCCMH, 2006:10.
[447] NCCMH, 2006:20.
[448] Fast & Preston, 2012:230-231.
[449] Mondimore, 1999:103.
[450] Haycock, 2010:74.
[451] Suppes & Keck, 2005:9.9.

proven especially effective for BP when combined with a mood stabiliser.[452] SSRIs are now preferred to Tricyclic Antidepressants (TCAs) and Monoamine Oxidase Inhibitors (MAOIs) because they are often just as effective and have a far superior side effect profile (they have fewer and less severe side effects).[453]

Some examples of SSRIs are: fluoxetine, sertraline, paroxetine and fluvoxamine.[454]

One thing that is vitally important to know about SSRIs is that they <u>must not</u> be taken at the same time as or within 14 days of an MAOI because this can cause dangerous reactions.[455]

MAOIs:

Monoamine Oxidase Inhibitors, or MAOIs, were initially used in the 1950s to treat tuberculosis when it was noticed to improve mood and even cause mania in some patients, so started to be used as an antidepressant.[456] Monoamine oxidase is an enzyme found in the brain 'that has been linked with depression'.[457] This is probably because it is 'responsible for gobbling up molecules of norepinephrine, serotonin and several other neurotransmitters'.[458] Because MAOIs block the activity of this enzyme, they increase the concentrations of norepinephrine and serotonin in the brain.[459] MAOIs 'appear to be superior to TCAs in their antidepressant activity in bipolar depression',[460] but their side effect profile is worse.

---

[452] Suppes & Keck, 2005:9.10
[453] Suppes & Keck, 2005:9.9; Mondimore, 1999:103.
[454] Haycock, 2010:74; Owen & Saunders, 2008:81; Mondimore, 1999:104.
[455] Shabbir et al., 2013; Evans & Allen, 2009:215.
[456] Mondimore, 1999:105.
[457] Haycock, 2010:74.
[458] Mondimore, 1999:105.
[459] Duke & Hochman, 1993:167.
[460] Suppes & Keck, 2005:9.17.

Examples of MAOIs include: phenelzine, nefazodone, tranylcypromine and isocarboxazid.[461]

However, MAOIs are now rarely used for treatment in bipolar unless other ADs simply do not work.[462] This is in part because the 'risk for developing mania is high'.[463] But it is mostly due to MAOIs' dangerous reaction with tyramine, which is found in a large number of foods and medications.[464] All food and medication containing tyramine must be strictly avoided if you are taking an MAOI (lists can easily be found on the internet).

You must also not take a TCA at the same time as an MAOI.[465] And again, please note: do not take an MAOI at the same time as an SSRI.[466]

TCAs:

Tricyclic Antidepressants, or TCAs, affect the activity of serotonin and norepinephrine.[467] Its main action is to inhibit the reuptake or reabsorbing of norepinephrine. This action led to early "amine theory" of bipolar disorder: that depression meant not enough norepinephrine and mania meant too much.[468]

It has been estimated that as many as 70% of bipolar depressed people may benefit from taking a TCA 'if they can tolerate the annoying, though not serious, side effects'.[469] However, treatment with TCAs should be alongside a mood stabiliser because TCAs are 'accompanied by a higher risk of manic or hypomanic switch' than

---

[461] Haycock, 2010:74; Duke & Hochman, 1993:167.
[462] Suppes & Keck, 2005:9.17; Mondimore, 1999:106.
[463] Suppes & Keck, 2005:9.17.
[464] Haycock, 2010:74; Evans & Allen, 2009:176; Mondimore, 1999:106.
[465] Evans & Allen, 2009:215.
[466] Shabbir et al., 2013.
[467] Haycock, 2010:75.
[468] Mondimore, 1999:100-101.
[469] Duke & Hochman, 1993:168.

other ADs.[470] TCAs are now only usually prescribed as a second or third course, if SSRIs are not well tolerated.[471] However, TCAs are particularly good at addressing treatment-resistant depression.[472]

Examples of TCAs include: imipramine, amitrityline, nortriptyline, desipramine and lofepramine.[473]

Do not take a TCA is you are also taking an MAOI, have had recent myocardial infarction, or have renal or hepatic disease.[474]

SNRIs:

Selective-Noradrenalin Reuptake Inhibitors, or SNRIs, are a relatively new class of antidepressant, as such I have found little research relating to their use in bipolar disorder. They work by blocking the reuptake of norepinephrine (also known as noradrenalin). Noradrenalin is one of the neurotransmitters where there seems to be a deficit during depression.

One example of an SNRI is venlafaxine. Though it is associated with lower risk of manic switch than TCAs,[475] it is not often prescribed because preliminary evidence suggests that 'compared with other equally effective antidepressants recommended for routine use in primary care, venlafaxine is associated with a greater risk of death by suicide'.[476]

Again, do not take an SNRI at the same time as an MAOI.[477]

AD side effects:

---

[470] Suppes & Keck, 2005:9.14.
[471] Haycock, 2010:75.
[472] Owen & Saunders, 2008:82.
[473] Haycock, 2010:75; Mondimore, 1999:102; Duke & Hochman, 1993:168.
[474] Evans & Allen, 2009:215.
[475] Owen & Saunders, 2008:81.
[476] NICE, 2014:24.
[477] Fast & Preston, 2012:230-231.

Of the antidepressants, SSRIs have the most 'favourable side effect profile'[478] with the most common side effects being insomnia, nausea, and vertigo (dizziness).[479] Though there is some evidence that sexual dysfunction may also be more common than originally thought.[480]

Aside from the very dangerous risk of 'blood pressure elevations unless certain foods and medications are avoided'[481] MAOIs have a host of mild to moderate side effects, including, but not limited to: sleep disturbances, dizziness, dry mouth, blurred vision, weight gain, constipation and the risk of hypomania.[482]

TCAs most serious, but uncommon, side effect is heart failure, or myocardial infarction. Other more common and less life-threatening side effects are: dry mouth, blurred vision, increased or decreased libido (sex drive), difficulty urinating, weight gain, constipation, and the more dangerous risk of mania.[483]

There is still not much information on the side effects of SNRIs.

"Switching":

Switching refers to an antidepressant-induced sudden change from depression to hypomania or mania, or an antidepressant-induced cycle acceleration from the person's regular course of illness to rapid cycling bipolar. There is a substantial body of evidence showing that monotherapy with ADs (taking an antidepressant alone) in people with bipolar disorder can cause switching,[484] either

---

[478] Suppes & Keck, 2005:9.9.
[479] Evans & Allen, 2009:215.
[480] Mondimore, 1999:104.
[481] Duke & Hochman, 1993:167.
[482] Evans & Allen, 2009:215; Duke & Hochman, 1993:167.
[483] Evans & Allen, 2009:215-216; Duke & Hochman, 1993:168.
[484] Hall-Flavin, 2012; Evans & Allen, 2009:159; NCCMH, 2006:10; Mondimore, 1999:100 & 107.

to (hypo)mania,[485] or to rapid cycling.[486] TCAs and MAOIs have been shown to have a higher switch rate than SSRIs; and TCA switches to be more intense.[487]

However, if treatment is combined with a mood stabiliser the risk of switching drops exponentially, perhaps as low as 5%-10%.[488] Be that as it may, recommendations are that those with bipolar do not continue on antidepressant treatment in the long term,[489] and if a person becomes hypomanic whilst being treated with an antidepressant, the AD should be stopped as quickly as possible.[490] However, as previously mentioned, since those of us with BPII spend more than 50% of our time depressed, it is not uncommon for us to take ADs long term provided it is with a mood stabiliser and closely monitored.[491] Despite the risks 'antidepressant medications have become very important in the treatment of bipolar disorder'.[492]

Anxiolytics:

Benzodiazepines, colloquially known as benzos, are part of a group of medications known as Central Nervous System (CNS) depressants.[493] CNS depressants work on neurotransmitters to slow down brain function. This is why they are used to treat anxiety, sleep disorders, hypomania and mania.[494]

Examples of benzodiazepines include: Alprazolam, Clonzepam,

---

[485] Fast & Preston, 2012:36 & 228; Hodges, 2012:31; Kennard, 2011:11; Marohn, 2011:56; Jackel, 2010; Myers & Thase, 2000; Boerlin et al., 1998.
[486] Ghaemi, 2008; McManamy, 2006:245; Zaretsky et al., 1999; Wehr & Goodwin, 1979.
[487] Boerlin et al., 1998.
[488] Haycock, 2010:73; Suppes & Keck, 2005:9.9-9.110; Thase & Sachs, 2000.
[489] NCCMH, 2006:10.
[490] NICE, 2014:21.
[491] Roberts et al., 2013:16.
[492] Mondimore, 1999:100.
[493] Fieve, 2006:191.
[494] Fieve, 2006:191.

Lorazepam, Diazepam and Propanol.[495]

Benzos are used to effectively treat the symptoms of anxiety by 'decreasing vigilance' and easing symptoms like muscle tension.[496] In an acute hypomanic episode, benzodiazepines may be prescribed to calm the person; by slowing down manic agitation benzos can literally be life-saving.[497] However, because of their addictive nature, these drugs are best only used for short term treatment of acute episodes of illness.[498]

You should not take a benzodiazepine if you are: under the influence of alcohol, pregnant or breast feeding, or have taken an MAOI antidepressant within the last 14 days.

Other meds:

Other medications which may be used at the prescriber's discretion to treat symptoms of BPII are sedatives (sleeping tablets).[499]

Knowledge:

Medication can literally save lives,[500] but that doesn't mean we should blindly accept everything the psychiatrist gives us. Knowledge is important. Before you start taking a medication it is recommended that you find out everything you can about it,[501] at the very least you should know the basics.[502] When you are prescribed any new medication the psychiatrist should: explain why they wish to put you on this med, give you a fact sheet or some

---

[495] Owen & Saunders, 2008:83; Fieve, 2006:191-193; Mondimore, 1999:117.
[496] Evans & Allen, 2009:196; Mondimore, 1999:116.
[497] NCCMH, 2006:17 & 207; Mondimore, 1999:117.
[498] NICE, 2011:18; Evans & Allen, 2009:196; Owen & Saunders, 2008:83; Fieve, 2006:191; NCCMH, 2006:207; Mondimore, 1999:116.
[499] Fletcher, 2017.
[500] Todd, 2016:22.
[501] Haycock, 2010:30.
[502] Fast & Preston, 2012:37.

other written information, give you the opportunity to ask questions, and take your opinion into account.

Side effects:

Some people say that side effects are an inevitable aspect of taking medications,[503] I disagree. All meds may have side effects, it's true,[504] but there is 'no such thing as a fair trade off' between improved BP symptoms and a worsened quality of life or the development of poor health.[505] The most challenging part of creating a medication regimen is finding a good balance between benefits and side effects. However, you do not have to tolerate any side effect that makes you feel unwell or unhappy. So try the meds with an open mind,[506] but always report any side effects straight away[507] or else your psychiatrist or GP cannot be expected to help you. If you experience intolerable side effects, your psychiatrist should offer to change your medication. It is important that, unless unavoidable, any psychiatric meds be discontinued gradually to reduce the risk of withdrawal symptoms.[508] If you experience problems, you and your doctor should only change one thing at a time (a change in dose or trying a new med) so that you can keep track of efficacy and side effects.[509]

So what should you look out for?

Each class of medication, and each medication in that class, has their own "side effect profile", some better than others. For example TCAs often have more side effects than SSRIs, and the reason most psychiatrists now use atypical/newer generation

---

[503] Kennard, 2011:17.
[504] White, 2014:73.
[505] McManamy, 2006:310.
[506] Fast & Preston, 2012:41.
[507] NIMH, 2018; White, 2014:73.
[508] Guyol, 2006:21; NCCMH, 2006:202 & 340.
[509] Haycock, 2010:78.

antipsychotics is because they have a far superior side effect profile to the typical/older generation antipsychotics of the 1950s and '60s.

I am not a fear monger, so I'm not going to give you a list of every side effect you could possibly get from BP meds. When you are prescribed any medication it comes with a comprehensive information sheet in the box that includes all the known potential side effects. It is important to emphasise the 'potential'; pharmaceutical companies have to list every possible side effect discovered during their extensive clinical trials for each drug. Usually the side effects section on these information sheets is graded from common to extremely rare. I recommend reading the info sheet thoroughly, but if you get a stomach ache that lasts a couple of days don't immediately assume you've developed stomach ulcers.

I'm going to focus on a few of the more common or least tolerable of the known side effects of BPII medications.

First, because lithium is so commonly prescribed for bipolar disorder, lithium toxicity must be covered; it is one of the most dangerous side effects we will discuss. If your lithium blood concentration gets too high this can cause irreparable damage to your vital systems. So, it is important to maintain a consistent intake of fluids and salt (don't drink 10 pints of water one day then just 1 the next) and it is integral that you always book and attend your lithium level blood tests, which should be every three to six months, or if you fall ill.

Next, the most common and intolerable side effect of a lot of BPII medications is rapid weight gain. An awful lot of bipolar meds cause weight gain.[510] It can be really distressing to find that a medication

---

[510] Paquette, 2016; White, 2014:75; Fast & Preston, 2012:40; Hall-Flavin, 2012; Hodges, 2012:74-77; Owen & Saunders, 2008:88; Guyol, 2006:18; McManamy, 2006:162; Mondimore, 1999:90-91.

that is helping with your mood symptoms has caused you to gain 10kg (22lb) in two months. In fact, this can have such a negative impact on mood that it counteracts the good being done by the medication. If you find you cannot tolerate the weight gain, make an emergency appointment to see your psychiatrist or GP; don't let rapid weight gain become a trigger for a depressive episode.

A frequently worried about, but thankfully uncommon, side effect is sexual dysfunction, particularly with SSRIs.[511] If you experience this side effect and it makes you unhappy make it known to your psychiatrist at your next appointment; it is not an emergency, but it does need to be sorted. If you find you experience sexual problems, but this is not an issue for you, great, but still point it out to your psychiatrist so they know.

Two side effects which may seem intolerable are insomnia and drowsiness.[512] If your med is otherwise working for you, simply ask your psychiatrist if you can change the timing of your dose(s); if it causes insomnia, take it in the morning, if it causes drowsiness, take it before bed.

A couple of other common, but quite manageable side effects are:[513]

- Dry mouth: drink plenty and eat mints or chew gum to keep your mouth moist.
- Stomach complaints: ask your GP for a stomach lining tablet to take in the morning, something like omeprazole.
- Constipation: take Senna every day, and if it gets really bad ask your GP for a laxative such as Laxido or Movicol.

---

[511] Fast & Preston, 2012:41; Guyol, 2006:17; McManamy, 2006:210-212.
[512] Fast & Preston, 2012:41; Dawson, 2006; Guyol, 2006:18; McManamy, 2006:210-212.
[513] Paquette, 2016; Hall-Flavin, 2012; Hodges, 2012:74-77; Guyol, 2006:17-18; McManamy, 2006:210-212; Mondimore, 1999:90-91.

- Headaches: drink plenty of water, get enough sleep and avoid caffeine.

Finally, one major side effect that can be very dangerous can sometimes occur in the first few weeks of antidepressant treatment. That is an increase in depressive symptoms, in particular suicidal and self-harm thoughts.[514] Of course, if you get a worsening of depressive symptoms and especially if you begin to feel suicidal, make an emergency appointment to see your psychiatrist and either go to A&E or go straight to your psychiatrist's clinic to see the duty worker (who is usually a psychiatric nurse or social worker).

Compliance:

Medication compliance, or adherence, means taking your prescriptions as intended; in the right doses, at the right times. However, almost half of those of us prescribed psychiatric meds do not take them properly.[515] More than half of patients experience some sort of side effects and nearly that number subsequently quit their meds.[516] People with bipolar may decide that the adverse effects simply outweigh the benefits.[517] It is vitally important that you never stop a medication without first talking with your psychiatrist; your body and brain will have gotten used to having the drug in your system and any sudden changes can cause serious and even dangerous effects.[518]

However, poor compliance is not just about not taking your meds; it's also non-compliance if you take more or less of a medication than instructed, if you take you medications at the wrong time, and also if you take it at the same time as substances you shouldn't be

---

[514] Guyol, 2006:20.
[515] Kennard, 2011:18.
[516] Fast & Preston, 2012:40; Haycock, 2010:109; Guyol, 2006:2 & 19.
[517] White, 2014:14-17; NCCMH, 2006:201 & 281.
[518] Todd, 2016:47; Chellingsworth & Farrand, 2015:49; White, 2014:13; Guyol, 2006:214; NCCMH, 2006:201.

taking (this could be using illicit drugs or it could be as simple as eating grapefruit).[519] Substance abuse, be it alcohol, over-the-counter medications or street drugs, is one of the most important risk factors for non-adherence in those with BPII.[520]

Another common reason for people not taking their meds is because they become hypomanic and feel that they no longer need them.[521]

Other reasons for non-compliance may be:[522]

- Stigma: there is still a certain stigma to taking medications for your mind,[523] but my argument is that there is greater stigma attached to going bankrupt, cheating on a partner, or ending up in jail/prison.
- Lack of understanding: the instructions given to the patient may not have been clear.
- The depressed person thinks their meds are not working: because you can still get depressed whilst on an AD, it is not unreasonable that the depressed mind, which already views things in their most negative light, might assume that their meds are not working so not see the point in taking them.
- Being forgetful: a person might simply be really bad at remembering to take their tablets.[524] If you have this problem, set reminders on your phone and keep your meds somewhere you'll see them every day, preferably in a dosette box.

Problems with non-compliance

---

[519] White, 2014:13.
[520] Jónsdóttir et al., 2012.
[521] Roberts et al., 2013:127.
[522] White, 2014:14-17.
[523] Todd, 2016:46.
[524] NCCMH, 2006:201.

In one study it was found that 23.6% of bipolar participants were non-compliant over the 21-month trial. The problems that arose from this non-adherence include: 'decreased likelihood of achieving remission and recovery as well as an increased risk of relapse and recurrence as well as hospitalization and suicide attempts'.[525] Non-compliance was generally associated with poorer outcomes over the course of illness, unsurprisingly.

Psychology & Psychotherapy
What is psychotherapy?

Psychotherapies are psychological interventions designed specifically to help people with mental health problems (everything ranging from stress to schizophrenia) to address challenges and help overcome problems related to their condition. Psychotherapy is not about a therapist, or psychologist, telling us what to do; it is about helping us to develop sensible, workable coping strategies to address our everyday issues;[526] it is about 'providing good information, objective feedback and solid encouragement';[527] and it is about learning about our illness,[528] all in a confidential and supportive setting.

Over recent years a number of psychotherapies have been developed or adapted specifically to treat bipolar.[529] The main aims of these psychological interventions are: 'the prevention of relapses and the promotion of social functioning ... the reduction of mood symptoms and mood fluctuations, promoting good coping skills, the enhancement of medication compliance and promoting communication within the family'.[530] Different psychotherapies have slightly different focuses. The four main types used to help

---

[525] Hong et al., 2011.
[526] Fieve, 2006:236.
[527] Mondimore, 1999:133-134.
[528] APA, 2017; Owen & Saunders, 2008:63; NCCMH, 2006:27.
[529] Otto et al., 2003.
[530] NCCMH, 2006:355.

treat BP are: Cognitive Behavioural Therapy (CBT), Family-Focused Therapy (FFT), Interpersonal and Social Rhythm Therapy (IPSRT) and Psychoeducation (PE);[531] though other therapies that may be offered include: Dialectal Behavioural Therapy (DBT), Mindfulness-Based Cognitive Therapy (MBCT), psychoanalysis and counselling.

So why do psychotherapy?

Typically people with BP are offered a psychotherapy referral by our psychiatrist or GP, and in my opinion we should utilise any help we can get in living and coping with our bipolar. On its own psychotherapy has been shown to be as effective as medication alone in the treatment of bipolar.[532] However, psychotherapy for BP is generally designed to be in addition to meds. An abundance of evidence supports that psychological interventions with medications greatly enhances outcomes for those with BP.[533] Psychotherapy has also been shown to improve medication compliance.[534] Psychological interventions have 'a proven track record in helping with depression'.[535] And it reduces the number of hospitalisations due to relapse.[536]

CBT:

Cognitive Behavioural Therapy, or CBT, is widely recommended by the NHS and NICE to address depression, particularly in bipolar.[537] This is mainly because CBT plus medications greatly improves the

---

[531] NIMH, 2018; Haycock, 2010:88; NCCMH, 2006:356.

[532] Guyol, 2006:13; Lam et al., 2005; Mondimore, 1999:133.

[533] NIMH, 2018; Haycock, 2010:93; Owen & Saunders, 2008:62; Miklowitz et al., 2007a; Miklowitz et al., 2007b; Bauer et al., 2006; Frank et al., 2006; Suppes & Keck, 2005:11.4; Duke & Hochman, 1993:176.

[534] Haycock, 2010:93; Miklowitz et al., 2007b; Duke & Hochman, 1993:177.

[535] Mondimore, 1999:137.

[536] Haycock, 2010:93.

[537] NHS, 2016; Chellingsworth & Farrand, 2015:34; NICE, 2009:11.

course of bipolar overall[538] and partly because it improves meds compliance.[539]

The main concept behind CBT is that our thoughts, moods, emotions and behaviours are all interconnected and influence each other.[540] As such, in CBT we learn the tools we need to change our thoughts and/or behaviours, in order to have a positive impact on our individual emotions and overall mood.[541] In particular, in CBT we focus on negative thoughts & perceptions, and cognitive distortions, such as all-or-nothing thinking or 'should' statements.[542] CBT also focuses on us changing our behaviours to promote healthier mood.[543]

There are plenty of resource books around which focus on CBT techniques; the one I most highly recommend for BPII is 'The Bipolar II Disorder Workbook' (Roberts et al., 2013), in particular pages 67-76, which are filled with useful and effective CBT exercises.

FFT:

Family-Focused Therapy, or FFT, was developed by David Miklowitz and Michael Goldstein in 1997.[544] It was borne out of the theory that a difficult or negative home environment increased the likelihood of bipolar relapse.[545] As such FFT involves the person with

---

[538] Barlow et al., 2016; Railton, 2016; Roberts et al., 2013:19; Kennard, 2011:20; Haycock, 2010:89; Ball et al., 2006; NCCMH, 2006:25; Lam et al., 2005; Zaretsky et al., 1999.
[539] Suppes & Keck, 2005:11.7; Cochran, 1984.
[540] Roberts et al., 2013:19; Haycock, 2010:88; Owen & Saunders, 2008:63.
[541] Roberts et al., 2013:67-76; Owen & Saunders, 2008:63; Teasdale et al., 2000; Duke & Hochman, 1993:179.
[542] Roberts et al., 2013:18 & 67; Haycock, 2010:88-89; Owen & Saunders, 2008:63; Miklowitz et al., 2007a; Fieve, 2006:240; Frank et al., 2006; NCCMH, 2006:357-358; Suppes & Keck, 2005:11.4.
[543] Chellingsworth & Farrand, 2015:37-38; Duke & Hochman, 1993:179.
[544] Roberts et al., 2013:18.
[545] Frank et al., 2006; Suppes & Keck, 2005:11.3.

bipolar and at least one family member or other person they live with.[546] The main aims are psychoeducation (teaching about bipolar), communication training, and problem-solving to address conflicts, misunderstandings and issues in the home.[547]

FFT in combination with pharmacotherapy (meds) has been shown to have a positive impact on bipolar in reducing stress, reducing the number of mood recurrences (by a factor of 28% to 35%), decreasing the number of hospitalisations, improving meds adherence and hastening recovery from current mood episodes.[548]

If you feel you may have interpersonal conflicts or misunderstandings among your family as a result of your bipolar, ask your psychiatrist for a referral for FFT. You may find that it helps. If nothing else it may help your family to be less confused about your condition.

IPSRT:

Interpersonal and Social Rhythm Therapy, or IPSRT, was designed by Ellen Frank in 2005.[549] IPSRT is focused on two main areas: interpersonal relationships & interactions, and daily routine & circadian rhythms.

When it comes to interpersonal relationships there are things to take into account: conflict, social anxiety and perceived ineptitude can cause a great deal of stress. This stress may be temporary or it may be long-lasting. And stress is bad for BPII. IPSRT explores the relationship between social interactions and mood[550] and helps us

---

[546] Haycock, 2010:91; Miklowitz et al., 2007a; Frank et al., 2006.
[547] NHS, 2016; Roberts et al., 2013:21; Haycock, 2010:91; Owen & Saunders, 2008:69; Miklowitz et al., 2007a; NCCMH, 2006:27; Suppes & Keck, 2005:1.3; Mondimore, 1999:141.
[548] Roberts et al., 2013:22; Haycock, 2010:91; Miklowitz et al., 2008; Suppes & Keck, 2005:11.5; Miklowitz, 2000; Duke & Hochman, 1993:176-177.
[549] Roberts et al., 2013:18.
[550] Miklowitz et al., 2007a; NCCMH, 2006:358; Suppes & Keck, 2005:11.4.

develop strategies to overcome conflict, improve our relationships and increase social functioning.[551]

Daily routine includes sleep/wake cycles, eating times and scheduling of activities. The aim of IPSRT in this area is to help us to establish a regular, stable routine.[552] The reasoning behind it is that disrupted daily rhythm, in particular irregular sleep, can lead to depressive or hypomanic episodes in those with BPII (more later).[553] So by establishing and maintaining a regular schedule, we are preventing bipolar episodes.

PE:

Psychoeducation, or PE, was fully developed in 2006 by a group of researchers in Spain.[554] The main purpose of Psychoeducation is to teach people with bipolar disorder about their condition and related relevant information.[555] Topics that may be covered include: recognition of bipolar prodromes (early warning signs), the benefits and risks of medication, tips for lifestyle regularity and stability, how to create mood diaries and the development of prevention programmes.

PE can be conducted individually, but is usually applied within a group setting. In this way not only can the psychotherapist provide information, but the attendees (all of whom will probably have an affective disorder) can share information and help each other

---

[551] Roberts et al., 2013:18; Haycock, 2010:89; Fieve, 2006:241; NCCMH, 2006:358; Duke & Hochman, 1993:176.
[552] Roberts et al., 2013:22; Haycock, 2010:89; Miklowitz et al., 2007a; Frank et al., 2006; NCCMH, 2006:358; Suppes & Keck, 2005:1.4; Mondimore, 1999:141.
[553] Roberts et al., 2013:22; Haycock, 2010:89; Miklowitz et al., 2007a; Frank et al., 2006; Ehlers et al., 1988.
[554] Roberts et al., 2013:18 & 23; Haycock, 2010:91.
[555] NHS, 2016; Roberts et al., 2013:23; Owen & Saunders, 2008:70; Frank et al., 2006; NCCMH, 2006:358 & 393; Suppes & Keck, 2005:11.1-11.2; Colom et al., 2003; Perry et al., 1999.

too.[556]

Psychoeducation has been shown to improve the course of illness for many people with BPII, especially for depressive symptoms.[557] Again, the best results come when PE is used to treat bipolar at the same time as meds.

DBT:

Dialectal Behavioural Therapy, or DBT, is similar to CBT in that they are both goal-oriented and focus a great deal on behaviour, but it has one key difference: in DBT you are supposed to recognise and accept 'overwhelming or painful emotions, without necessarily trying to change [them]'.[558]

The most striking feature of DBT is that, in comparison to other therapies, it has the best reputation for reducing or alleviating suicidal thoughts, ideation and attempts.[559]

MBCT:

Mindfulness-Based Cognitive Therapy, or MBCT, was designed as a group approach, rather than for individuals. It was created to treat unipolar depressed people who had recurrent episodes, and it proved quite effective.[560] The theory of mindfulness is explored later in more detail, but in short, in MBCT rather than confront your negative thoughts and emotions, you notice them, accept them and move past them in 'healthier, or less negative, ways'[561] viewing them as "mental acts" rather than as 'aspects of the self or as

---

[556] Owen & Saunders, 2008:70; Mondimore, 1999:136-137.
[557] Roberts et al., 2013:23; Haycock, 2010:91; Bauer et al., 2006; NCCMH, 2006:392; Colom et al., 2003; Perry et al., 1999.
[558] Roberts et al., 2013:20; Fieve, 2006:240.
[559] Roberts et al., 2013:20; Goldstein et al., 2007; Linehan et al., 2006.
[560] Roberts et al., 2013:21; Teasdale, 2000.
[561] Roberts et al., 2013:21.

necessarily accurate reflections of reality'.[562]

In bipolar, unfortunately, MBCT does not seem to have the same effect as with unipolar depression. However, it is still useful. Treatment with MBCT between mood episodes has been shown to have positive effects on residual mood symptoms[563] and a marked impact on the prevalence of anxiety symptoms or comorbid anxiety disorders.[564]

Others:

Talk therapy or counselling may prove useful, in particular for those who have difficulties with meds compliance.[565]

Psychoanalysis "digs" into past traumas, so may prove useful if you have issues which have arisen from bipolar behaviours or if you have PTSD.[566]

The future of therapy:

Psychotherapy has come a long way in the past couple of decades, but there is always room for improvement. At the moment the 'availability of services varies tremendously by area',[567] it may be that you are on the waiting list for over a year even in NHS localities where psychotherapy is available for referral, and not all localities have psychologists or therapists so you may have to travel a fair way. Alternatively you can go private, and many people do.

In terms of the psychotherapies currently on the market, more research is being undertaken on CBT following recommendations[568]

---

[562] Teasdale, 2000.
[563] Deckersbach et al., 2012.
[564] Perich et al., 2013; Roberts et al., 2013:21.
[565] McManamy, 2006:260.
[566] Duke & Hochman, 1993:179.
[567] Chellingsworth & Farrand, 2015:48.
[568] Zaretsky et al., 1999.

and new strategies for PE are being applied all the time.[569]

Some researchers, however, want to see the construction of new 'hybrid models of psychotherapy', incorporating the most successful aspects of the various strategies.[570] And I think this is indeed the future.

Complementary and Alternative Medicine

Complementary and alternative medicine (CAM), also known as natural medicine,[571] is the practice of using non-pharmaceutical treatments for various medical conditions. There are a range of CAMs available which are used by holistic practitioners and healers across the UK to treat bipolar. Including, but not limited to: aromatherapy, massage, chiropractic treatment, acupuncture, herbal teas, homeopathic remedies, and naturopathy.[572] The theory is that CAMs 'operate according to holistic principles',[573] that is, they aim to treat the whole person rather than targeting the symptoms individually.

However, it is worth noting that "natural" does not automatically mean "safe"[574] for example St John's Wort interacts with a number of medications and other supplements with dangerous effects.[575] And other supplements when taken together with certain medications 'may cause unwanted or dangerous effects'.[576] So you should always talk with your psychiatrist before starting any CAM[577] and even the majority of holistic practitioners advise that you should not reduce or stop your psychiatric meds without seeking

---

[569] Lam & Wong, 1997.
[570] Miklowitz et al., 2007b.
[571] Marohn, 2011:xiv.
[572] Fast & Preston, 2012:73.
[573] Marohn, 2011:xiii.
[574] Fast & Preston, 2012:73; McManamy, 2006:278.
[575] Fast & Preston, 2012:236; Haycock, 2010:99.
[576] NIMH, 2018.
[577] Hodges, 2012:82.

help from your psychiatrist as 'any sudden change may cause serious reactions and endanger your health'.[578] And nearly all medical scientists recommend that 'people with psychiatric disorders should not rely on alternative treatments to the exclusion of established therapies'.[579]

That being said many complementary and alternative therapies are quite safe and, if they are, may provide some benefit, even if it is simply to induce relaxation.[580] Many people with BPII find that incorporating some holistic practices into their treatment plan helps them to 'control symptoms and prolong periods of stability'.[581] In particular many CAMs are excellent stress-busters.[582] Though, as with pharmacology and psychotherapy, the benefits of CAM may take a while to become apparent as most are targeted at helping the body to 'repair and rebuild [its] own systems'.[583]

Supplements:

There is a plethora of literature suggesting that the use of various supplements (neutraceuticals) may help in the management of bipolar, or at least its symptoms. It has been suggested that in addition to medications 'treatment outcomes may potentially be improved by the additional use of certain neutraceuticals'.[584] These include but are not limited to: omega-3 fatty acids (omega-3 PUFA), magnesium, SAM-e, tryptophan, taurine, vitamin D, amino acids, and methionine.[585]

There is some evidence to support the use of supplements as an

---

[578] Guyol, 2006:214.
[579] Haycock, 2010:243.
[580] Haycock, 2010:243.
[581] Owen & Saunders, 2008:184.
[582] Wilkinson, 1999:82.
[583] Guyol, 2006:220.
[584] Sarris et al., 2011.
[585] Railton, 2016; Hodges, 2012:85-87; Khamba et al., 2011; Marohn, 2011:41-43; Guyol, 2006:217-218; McManamy, 2006:285; Beckham, 1983.

adjunct treatment or self-management technique for BP, but '[not] much research has been conducted in comparison to pharmaceuticals'[586] so they should not be considered as an alternative to meds, but an addition to. It is recommended that before you start on any specific regime of supplements you begin by 'taking high-quality vitamin/mineral supplements, fish oils, and perhaps amino acids'.[587] Again though, talk with your psychiatrist first to make sure there are no contraindications (reasons not to).

Magnesium

Magnesium deficiency has been linked with increased anxiety and irritability, symptoms of both hypomania and depression.[588] As such magnesium is sometimes recommended for its calming effect.[589]

Zinc

Low zinc levels have been linked to apathy, loss of appetite and lethargy, all symptoms of depression.[590]

Tyrosine

Tyrosine is a precursor (building block) of norepinephrine and dopamine.[591] As such it can be used to lift depression and may also aid in stress management[592] though too much can cause mania.[593]

Phenylalanine

Phenylalanine is one of the "trace amines" which may be 'out of

---

[586] NIMH, 2018.
[587] Guyol, 2006:216.
[588] Owen & Saunders, 2008:197.
[589] Railton, 2016; Marohn, 2011:43.
[590] Khamba et al., 2011; Haycock, 2010:85; Owen & Saunders, 2008:199.
[591] McManamy, 2006:285.
[592] Marohn, 2011:41; Guyol, 2006:217.
[593] Guyol, 2006:217.

order in depressed patients'[594] so might be useful in the treatment of bipolar depression.[595]

Taurine

Taurine is recommended for its calming qualities[596] which may help alleviate hypomanic symptoms.

Vitamin D

'Vitamin D is a steroid hormone that plays several important physiologic roles'[597] including regulation of mood and the promotion of sound sleep.[598] This is probably because vitamin D has been shown to stimulate serotonin production.[599]

Methionine

Methionine may be useful in the reduction of hypomanic and anxious symptoms.[600]

Vitamin B-complex

B-vitamins deficiency has been related to brain and behaviour disorders and lower response to antidepressants.[601] Low folate and vitamin B_{12} have been demonstrated to have 'adverse neuropsychiatric effects'[602] such as a connection with depression.[603] B_1 deficiency can lead to 'fatigue, depression, irritability, anxiety and even thoughts of suicide;'[604] B_3 deficiency can cause agitation and

---

[594] Beckham, 1983.
[595] Marohn, 2011:41; Guyol, 2006:217.
[596] Hodges, 2012:85-87; McManamy, 2006:285.
[597] Khamba et al., 2011.
[598] Hodges, 2012:85; Khamba et al., 2011.
[599] Khamba et al., 2011.
[600] Guyol, 2006:217-218.
[601] McManamy, 2006:283.
[602] Freeman et al., 2006.
[603] Hodges, 2012:83-85; Owen & Saunders, 2008:196.
[604] Owen & Saunders, 2008:197.

anxiety; B$_5$ deficiency has been linked to 'fatigue, chronic stress and depression'; B$_6$ helps to make serotonin; and B$_{12}$ is vital to a healthy nervous system.[605] Altogether, B-vitamins are vital to neurotransmitter function.[606]

Omega-3 Polyunsaturated Fatty Acids (PUFA)

A significant amount of research has been conducted on the effects of omega-3 on mood disorders; in particular the effects of EPA and DHA (the "active" elements of omega-3).

Most evidence shows that omega-3, or EPA & DHA, supplementation has a minor positive effect on bipolar depressive symptoms.[607] Though some of the evidence is mixed[608] and some studies show no or negligible effect.[609] However no studies have found any risk to taking omega-3 supplements and it may incur other health benefits.[610] However, as with other supplements, it is not recommended that those of us with BPII take omega-3 instead of medication, but rather as an addition to.[611]

SAM-e

SAM-e levels have been shown to be much lower in depressed people,[612] as such, SAM-e supplementation may reduce depression.[613] In fact, SAM-e has been used in Europe for over two

---

[605] Owen & Saunders, 2008:198.
[606] Marohn, 2011:42.
[607] White, 2014:67; Fast & Preston, 2012:235; Hodges, 2012:83-85; Marohn, 2011:39; Haycock, 2010:99; Liperoti et al., 2009; Owen & Saunders, 2008:199; Stahl et al., 2008; McManamy, 2006:287; Parker et al., 2006.
[608] Rogers et al., 2008.
[609] White, 2014:67; Liperoti et al., 2009; Rogers et al., 2008; Stahl et al., 2008; Freeman et al., 2006.
[610] Fast & Preston, 2012:235.
[611] Freeman et al., 2006.
[612] McManamy, 2006:290.
[613] Haycock, 2010:99.

decades to treat depression.[614] In a 2010 study, 36% of people taking a combination of SAM-e and an antidepressant 'showed improvement' and around 26% 'experienced complete remission of symptoms'.[615]

Again, it is recommended you speak to your psychiatrist before starting SAM-e supplements as it is well known to cause mania.[616]

St John's wort

St John's wort is sometimes recommended as a treatment for depression. It is NOT, however, recommended for bipolar disorder[617] or for those taking ANY medication as it has numerous drug interactions.[618]

Tryptophan/5-HTP

Tryptophan is a precursor (building block) of serotonin[619] and some researchers have found supplementation or a diet high in tryptophan to be beneficial in the reduction of bipolar depressive symptoms.[620] Though others have found tryptophan or 5-HTP alone to not be useful for bipolar depressed people, it has been suggested that tryptophan may 'potentiate the action of' tricyclic antidepressants (TCAs) in bipolar.[621] It is worth noting that too much tryptophan or 5-HTP 'may produce nausea, other gastrointestinal distress, and drowsiness'.[622]

GABA

---

[614] Fast & Preston, 2012:236.
[615] Hodges, 2012:87.
[616] Fast & Preston, 2012:236; Hodges, 2012:87.
[617] Hodges, 2012:85-87; Owen & Saunders, 2008:201.
[618] Fast & Preston, 2012:236; Haycock, 2010:99.
[619] McManamy, 2006:285.
[620] White, 2014:70; Hodges, 2012:83; Marohn, 2011:41; Guyol, 2006:217, McManamy, 2006:285; Chouinard et al., 1983.
[621] Chouinard et al., 1983.
[622] Marohn, 2011:41.

Gamma-aminobutyric acid (GABA) has been described as "our natural Valium".[623] It is known to reduce stress and promote good sleep[624] and has also 'proven useful in the treatment of mania, acute agitation, anxiety, nervous tension, hyperactivity'.[625]

Valerian Root

It is not 'advisable to take Valerian Root alongside pharmaceutical medications'.[626] Though for those not on meds, valerian tea may help promote sleep.

Melatonin

Melatonin is one of the body's natural hormones which helps to regulate our sleep/wake cycle. Ideally our melatonin levels should be low in the morning and high in the evening because melatonin promotes tiredness.[627] However, melatonin seems to be incorrectly secreted in BP, '[not] only the levels but the timings of secretion are altered in bipolar disorder'.[628] Meaning that we have the wrong levels at the wrong times. This goes some way to explaining why sleep problems are so common in BP. If you find you have trouble sleeping, in particular getting off to sleep, instead of asking your GP or psychiatrist for sleeping pills, you might suggest melatonin tablets. You take them a couple of hours before you want to sleep, they cause no harm and the only usual side effect is drowsiness; if you have trouble sleeping, that's what you want.

light therapy:

---

[623] McManamy, 2006:285.
[624] Hodges, 2012:85-87; Guyol, 2006:217.
[625] Marohn, 2011:41.
[626] Hodges, 2012:85-87.
[627] Hodges, 2012:85-87.
[628] Srinivasan et al., 2006:

There is a treatment for depression known as light therapy, or bright light therapy, which is completely non-invasive and does not require you to take any tablets or supplements. In this therapy you need either a light box (available for as little as £50 for a good one) or a daylight bulb (available for as little as £9 on the internet, though not as effective as a light box). You use the light box for 10-30 minutes a day, depending on the recommendation of your psychiatrist, usually in the morning. You keep the light box turned on and well within your vision with your eyes open; just don't stare at it because this may strain or even hurt your eyes. You may choose to read or to write in your mood journal for the allotted time.

The way bright light therapy works is it suppresses the production of melatonin (a hormone that helps manage the sleep/wake cycle).[629] So not only is it an effective treatment for bipolar disorder in its own right, but it also helps you to feel more awake in the morning and more sleepy in the evening, helping you to get into a healthy, natural sleep/wake cycle.

A word of warning: The use of a light box can induce mania, so for the first couple of weeks of use it is vital that you carefully monitor your mood and behaviour for any signs or symptoms of hypomania.[630] If these occur, stop using your light box and make an appointment with your psychiatrist so they can help to judge your mood.

Massage:

Massage, also known as therapeutic touch, hands-on healing or gentle touch,[631] is one of the oldest healing techniques.[632] Massage

---

[629] Srinivasan et al., 2006.
[630] McManamy, 2006:291.
[631] Guyol, 2006:187-188.
[632] Owen & Saunders, 2008:185.

is used by modern medicine to relieve pain, aid in post-operative healing, and reduce stress and anxiety.[633] For some practitioners massage is intended to enhance the flow of energy 'in the body and aura',[634] but regardless of the intention, massage is a safe 'passive route to physical relaxation and stress relief'[635] and for many people with BPII, is one of the most beneficial CAM therapies.[636]

Acupuncture:

Clinical trials using acupuncture for bipolar depression have yielded inconclusive results,[637] however, in some studies as much as 43% of patients showed a reduction of depressive symptoms.

In acupuncture, a series of super-fine needles are placed along the 'energy lines', or meridians, of the body to help relieve medical conditions.[638] As with therapeutic touch, acupuncture is now used by Western medicine to relieve pain, aid in post-operative healing, and reduce stress and anxiety,[639] as well as to directly treat medical issues, including mental health disorders. The aim is to '[address] energy imbalances' and enhance the flow of energy through the 'body and aura'.[640]

Reiki:

Reiki is a treatment in which the practitioner uses their body, in particular their hands, to channel healing energy throughout the body of the client.[641] The practice comes from Japan, and reiki means 'universal spirit'. It is this universal energy that the

---

[633] Owen & Saunders, 2008:185; Guyol, 2006:190.
[634] Guyol, 2006:188.
[635] Haycock, 2010:100.
[636] Hodges, 2012:89.
[637] Guyol, 2006:192.
[638] Owen & Saunders, 2008:184.
[639] Guyol, 2006:190.
[640] Marohn, 2011:56; Guyol, 2006:188.
[641] Owen & Saunders, 2008:187.

practitioner channels into the clients body to precipitate healing.

Again, in modern Western medicine reiki is now used to alleviate stress and anxiety, among other things.[642] Reiki has been shown to have positive effects on depression.[643]

To learn more about reiki, I highly recommend the book 'Reiki for Life' by Penelope Quest, world-renowned reiki master.

Neurofeedback/Brain Biofeedback:

Neurofeedback, or brain biofeedback, is difficult to explain, but essentially my understanding of it is: you are wired up to two computer screens: one shows an EEG of your brain, the other a puzzle or video game for you to play. The concept is that certain tasks in the game promote the use of certain functions in your brain, so certain parts of your brain "light up" on the EEG and you get "rewards" when the right parts light up. After a while the aim is that you will be able to choose to light up these certain areas of your brain. The parts that are being "trained" are the calming centres of your brain, so when you can light them up yourself, you can reduce your anxiety.

Neurofeedback has been used as an adjunctive (additional) therapy for anxiety, depression and bipolar disorder, as well as other psychiatric conditions.[644] However, case studies on the treatment of BP with neurofeedback have produced mixed results.[645] That being said, neurofeedback is not harmful in any known way, so it may be worth giving it a try. And there is no evidence that you can't take your psychiatric meds and receive neurofeedback at the same

---

[642] Guyol, 2006:190.
[643] Guyol, 2006:192.
[644] Guyol, 2006:153; Oubr, 2002.
[645] Oubr, 2002.

time.[646]

Homeopathy:

In homeopathy, plants, minerals and other substances are distilled into water hundreds of times and the resulting product is a homeopathic remedy. The idea is not that the biological properties of the original substance, but rather the 'energetic patterns' remain intact, and the remedy seeks to transfer this energy to the person taking it.[647] The aim of homeopathy is to 'address energy imbalances'.[648] This is done through a holistic approach; considering the person as a whole, as an individual, and targeting the root of the problem.[649] Because homeopathic remedies in theory no longer contain any trace elements of their original substances, they are considered safe, do not have any side effects, and the effects become apparent after a single dose.[650]

Psychospiritual:

Because some holistic practitioners view bipolar as a partly spiritual condition it has been suggested that we '[e]xplore psychospiritual issues through psychotherapy or other modalities'[651] or through prayer.[652]

Other Complementary and Alternative Medicines:

Some other therapies used to treat bipolar disorder either independently or as an adjunct to psychotherapy or psychopharmacology include:

---

[646] Oubr, 2002.
[647] Marohn, 2011:158; Owen & Saunders, 2008:185.
[648] Marohn, 2011:56.
[649] Marohn, 2011:163.
[650] Marohn, 2011:163-164.
[651] Marohn, 2011:56.
[652] Guyol, 2006:182.

- orthomolecular treatments
- aromatherapy
- naturopathy
- other forms of energy healing
- Yoga
- nutrition (see section on 'Diet')
- chiropractic treatments.

For an excellent resource and much more thorough explanation of these and other natural medicines I highly recommend Stephanie Marohn's 'The Natural Medicine Guide to Bipolar Disorder'.[653]

Advanced Directives

In some cases, people with BPII are not in a fit state to make decisions about their psychiatric care,[654] for example if they are catatonic (non-responsive and disinterested) and suicidal during a depressive phase.[655] If there is a risk of this happening to you, then when you are creating your crisis plan with your psychiatrist or care co-ordinator,[656] you may wish to include an Advanced Directive. This is where you write down things you would or would not like to happen to/for you should you become incapacitated under the guidelines of the Mental Capacity Act. Things you can include should primarily be about your treatment. It might include where you would like to go if you require hospitalisation, which treatments or medications you do not want (for example if you had a negative reaction to a medication you tried in the past), which treatments you suggest may be beneficial, based on your experience, and who you would like to be involved in your care, like your CPN or social worker. Under the Mental Capacity Act, any treatments you DON'T want to have must be respected by law, however any requests you have made may be ignored if the mental health team deems them

---

[653] Marohn, 2011.
[654] NHS, 2016.
[655] Mondimore, 1999:238.
[656] NCCMH, 2006:11.

not to be in your best interest.[657] In your Advanced Directive you can give permission to someone in particular to make decisions about your care on your behalf,[658] this should be someone like a family member ideally. A copy of your crisis plan, and your Advanced Directive, should be given to you and another to your GP.[659] It is also recommended you provide a copy to your next of kin or carer.

---

[657] Owen & Saunders, 2008:103-104.
[658] Haycock, 2010:165.
[659] NCCMH, 2006:11.

Chapter Four:

Management and Lifestyle

Sleep

Sleep is vital to all good health.[660] Sleep disturbances are both symptoms and triggers of bipolar episodes.[661] Poor sleep is often a predicate to a mood episode, and a lot of evidence indicates that a lack of sleep often heralds an impending episode,[662] though it may just as easily be hypomania as depression; if nothing else it can lead to exhaustion.[663] Research shows that up to 80% of people with psychiatric disorders have sleep disorders.[664]

It seems people with BPII are especially 'sensitive to disruption in their sleep pattern'[665] and some suspect that we may be more susceptible to sleep 'abnormalities'.[666] During both depression and hypomania many people with BP report sleeping fewer than six hours a night,[667] though because bipolar depression is often characterised by 'atypical' features, sometimes we may sleep fourteen hours and still not feel rested. That's the big difference between sleep during depression and sleep during hypomania how tired we feel. When hypomanic we might sleep three hours and wake up feeling fresh as a daisy. When depressed we may sleep thirteen and still need a nap an hour after we get up. But even sleep variability when euthymic (normal mood) is associated with 'increased mania and depression severity'.[668]

Getting good sleep on the other hand, is both a way of preventing bipolar relapse and a way of identifying that you are less likely to be

---

[660] Railton, 2016; NCCMH, 2006:21; Perlman et al., 2006.
[661] White, 2014:41; Roberts et al., 2013:51; Haycock, 2010:63; Owen & Saunders, 2008:37 & 179; NCCMH, 2006:276 & 397; Perlman et al., 2006; Maas, 1999.
[662] APA, 2017; White, 2014:41; Baglioni et al., 2011; Marohn, 2011:50; Fieve, 2006:88; Wehr et al., 1987.
[663] Evans & Allen, 2009:153.
[664] Owen & Saunders, 2008:179.
[665] Kennard, 2011:23.
[666] Fieve, 2006:88.
[667] Perlman et al., 2006.
[668] Marohn, 2011:27; Gruber et al., 2011.

experiencing a mood episode.[669] If you find you are not sleeping or you're tired all the time, check your meds: some bipolar medications cause fatigue, others insomnia,[670] you may find it's worth talking to your doctor about timing for your doses.

So how do you increase your chances of good sleep?

Nothing you do can guarantee you a good, restful night's sleep, but using sleep hygiene techniques can greatly increase the chances.[671] To get your recommended 7-8 hours a night[672] here are some tips for you to try:

- Lavender on or under your pillow: lavender is relaxing, a couple of drops on your pillow or a small bunch underneath can be calming and aid sleep.
- Try to keep regular sleep/wake hours: wherever possible try to go to bed and get up at the same time every day, even on weekends.
- Make sure your bedroom is a restful environment: keep your room tidy, try to have your room dark and cool, and depending on which helps you sleep either make your room silent or play quiet music/ambient noise.
- Have a warm drink: ideally something without caffeine. Warm milk is ideal.
- Make sure your bed is comfy: you need to feel good when you lie down, try to have a mattress that is just right for you, pillows that are the right height to support your neck and head, and covers or a duvet that are the most comfortable weight for you.

---

[669] Todd, 2016:31; White, 2014:41.
[670] Dawson, 2006.
[671] NHS, 2018; White, 2014:45; Roberts et al., 2013:126; Baglioni et al., 2011; Miller, 2009:36 & 107 & 243; Owen & Saunders, 2008:180-181; Frank et al., 2006; McManamy, 2006:167-170; Srinivasan et al., 2006; Mondimore, 1999:226; Wilkinson, 1999:35-36.
[672] bipolarUK, 2018; Owen & Saunders, 2008:176.

- Drink less caffeine: a lot of people with and without bipolar choose not to drink caffeinated drinks (including cola) after a certain point in the afternoon, say four o'clock. Caffeine is a stimulant and may well keep you up.
- Exercise regularly: getting at least twenty minutes of moderate-intensity exercise each day has been proven to improve chances of a decent night's sleep. Exercise helps your body to become physically tired. However, don't do your exercise within the last couple of hours before you go to bed else the endorphins released will still be in your system and can keep you up.
- Don't binge: by all means have a light snack before bed (fruit or some cheese and crackers are a sound option), but the last big meal of the day should be at least three hours before bedtime.
- Don't smoke: nicotine is a stimulant, so a cigarette just before bed may well keep you up.
- Try to relax: just before bed do something calming and relaxing, such as having a bath or meditating. Try to avoid watching TV or surfing the net, staring at these screens can actually "switch you on" just before bed.
- Don't worry in bed: keep a regular to-do list and each evening write down what you have to do tomorrow. First it means you're less likely to forget, second, you're less likely to think about it in bed.
- If you can't sleep, get up: if you find you've been lying in bed for what feels like forever, but not sleeping, get up. Go read a book, do the dishes, meditate a while, then try again.
- Drink herbal tea: some herbal teas such as chamomile are especially relaxing and aid with sleep.
- If you find you have insomnia night after night go speak to your GP. They may be willing to prescribe you a short course of sleeping tablets to kick-start a healthy sleep pattern once more. It is best however to avoid taking sleeping tablets too many nights in a row as you can

become dependent. If insomnia persists, perhaps ask if you can try melatonin which is a hormone naturally secreted by the body to help manage our sleep wake cycles. It is best to take melatonin about an hour and a half before you want to sleep.
- If you find you are sleeping all the time and still feeling tired, you may well be at the start of a depressive episode. Get yourself to your psychiatrist and explain, they can prescribe you some antidepressants to nip it in the bud before it gets out of hand.

Hopefully these tips will help you get some rest and rejuvenation.

Stress

Stress can be really damaging in BPII. Even a seemingly trivial stressful situation, good or bad, can become overwhelming.[673] Stress can have devastating effects on mood,[674] and '[poor] stress management can exacerbate mental health conditions'.[675] As such it is recommended that people with bipolar try to avoid stress.[676] That being said, it is impossible to avoid all stress, and the best stress management in the world cannot always protect us.[677]

Stress is a trigger:

A trigger is any event or situation that directly precipitates a mood episode.[678] It is quite common for stressful life events to be triggers,[679] especially early in the course of illness.[680] Positive events as well as negative events can be triggers,[681] such as weddings or

---

[673] Fast & Preston, 2012:29.
[674] McManamy, 2006:107.
[675] Fletcher, 2017.
[676] bipolarUK, 2018.
[677] NCCMH, 2006:396.
[678] Fast & Preston, 2012:79.
[679] Todd, 2016:39; White, 2014:28; Hodges, 2012:16; Marohn, 2011:29; Johnson, 2005.
[680] Marohn, 2011:30.
[681] Owen & Saunders, 2008:177.

the birth of a child. Even small stresses like a sudden change in routine or a single bad night's sleep can be enough to set off a mood episode.[682] This is sometimes known as the 'diathesis-stress model'; essentially mental health conditions are influenced not only by our genes, but also by our environment and the stresses that come with it.[683]

What does stress do to us?

'Too much stress ... affects our health and well-being'.[684] Chronic stress 'wreaks havoc on the body, mind and spirit'.[685] Emotionally stress can cause depression, anxiety, irritability, frustration and anger[686] and has 'a weakening and demoralising effect'.[687] Physically it raises our cortisol levels (which can lead to depression),[688] and it puts strain on our nutrient absorbption and lowers our immunity[689] making us more prone to sicknesses such as colds and "tummy bugs".

Symptoms of stress:

The symptoms of stress vary from person to person, however, most of us have our own typical 'stress response'.[690]

The most comprehensive lists of symptoms come from Wilkinson, 1999, pages 17-19. Here they are:

- 'Emotional Reactions to Stress':[691]
    -Feeling under pressure,

---

[682] Frank et al., 2006.
[683] Roberts et al., 2013:17.
[684] Wilkinson, 1999:8.
[685] Marohn, 2011:29.
[686] Owen & Saunders, 2008:176.
[687] Wilkinson, 1999:8.
[688] Wooldridge, 2016:14.
[689] Marohn, 2011:29.
[690] Wilkinson, 1999:16.
[691] Wilkinson, 1999:17.

-Feeling tense and unable to relax,
-Feeling mentally drained,
-Being constantly frightened or worried,
-Increased irritability and complaining,
-Feeling of conflict,
-Frustration and aggression,
-Restlessness, increasing inability to concentrate or to complete tasks quickly,
-Increased tearfulness,
-Becoming more fussy, gloomy or suspicious,
-Being unable to take decisions,
-Impulses to run and hide,
-Fears of imminent fainting, collapse or death,
-Fears of social embarrassment or failure,
-Lacking in ability to feel pleasure.

- 'Physical Reactions to Stress':[692]
    -Muscle tension,
    -Rapid, uneven or pounding heartbeat,
    -Fast, shallow breathing,
    -Sweating,
    -Dilated pupils,
    -Over-alertness,
    -Change in appetite,
    -Muscle weakness or trembling,
    -A sick feeling in the stomach,
    -Sleep problems,
    -Jumpiness,
    -Headaches,
    -Weakness of the limbs,
    -Indigestion,
    -Frequent urge to pass urine,
    -Chest discomfort,
    -Odd aches, pains or twitches,
    -Constipation or diarrhoea,

---

[692] Wilkinson, 1999:18.

- Tiredness or weakness,
- Worsening of long-standing pain,
- Constant restlessness and fidgeting,
- Backache,
- 'Pins and needles',
- Dry mouth or throat,
- 'Butterflies' in the stomach.
* Long term reactions to stress:[693]
  - hair loss,
  - mouth ulcers,
  - asthma aggravation,
  - high blood pressure,
  - IBS,
  - indigestion,
  - irritable bladder.

Overcoming stress

In many circumstances, stress can be overcome or at least coped with in a healthy manner. When we know we can do this, stress becomes less of a trigger and less harmful.[694] Because of the above there is a 'strong argument for reducing the amount of stress in your life'.[695]

One of the easiest ways to reduce the amount of stress in your life is to simply avoid stressful situations;[696] this means you need to develop self-knowledge and awareness to accept your limitations.[697] However, it is not always possible, or indeed wise, to avoid all stressful situations. For example, you may choose not to work because job interviews and the work environment are too stressful. But if you do this you will then have to face regular

---

[693] Wilkinson, 1999:19.
[694] Boyes, 2015:30.
[695] Marohn, 2011:30.
[696] bipolar UK, 2018; Boyes, 2015:181; Kennard, 2011:27; Marohn, 2011:30.
[697] Haycock, 2010:188.

appointments at the Job Centre which may be just as stressful. Avoiding both will lead to your having no income from wages or benefits.

The best way to cope with stress is to shore up against it. That is to put preventative measures and anticipatory (forward-thinking) coping strategies in place. 'Lifestyle changes often make a huge difference in the reserves and resources people have available to cope with stress'.[698]

The first tip is to get in plenty of relaxation time, we all need time to rest and recuperate from both daily and larger life stresses.[699] The advantages of regular relaxation should not be underestimated: improved sleep, increased mental and physical performance, reduced tiredness, decreased tension and anxiety, and best of all, it is not addictive or prone to negative side effects.[700]

Some simple ways to manage stress may seem quite obvious once they're pointed out:

- Find the cause and try to address it.[701]
- Learn to say no: when you know you're taking on a lot, start to say no when asked to do other things too. Say no to that extra project at work, don't do that extra thing for someone else. Look after you.[702]
- Avoid always talking about your stress: focusing on it all the time will only make it worse.[703]

---

[698] Boyes, 2015:182; Kennard, 2011:27; Marohn, 2011:30; Wilkinson, 1999:26.
[699] Boyes, 2015:181; Marohn, 2011:30; Owen & Saunders, 2008:176; Wilkinson, 1999:40.
[700] Wilkinson, 1999:40.
[701] Miller, 2009:225; Wilkinson, 1999:9.
[702] Miller, 2009:225.
[703] Boyes, 2015:186-187.

- Talk to people: try to resolve stressful situations involving other people by having a conversation with them, even if they may try to guilt trip you.[704]
- Don't procrastinate: 'Putting off things until the last minute invariably raises stress levels'.[705]
- Go part-time: if you love your job, but it's stressful, see if you can go part-time or job-share.[706]
- Quit: if you have a stressful job you don't like, look for a new job.[707]

Exercise

Regular physical activity, or exercise, is widely recommended as a positive self-help technique for those of us with BPII,[708] especially when we are depressed.[709]

What is exercise?

The Oxford English Dictionary defines exercise as:

'activity requiring physical effort carried out for the sake of health and fitness.'

So exercise is the deliberate act of undertaking physical activity with the purpose of staying or getting fit and healthy.

There are three main classes of exercise: cardiovascular or aerobic exercise, muscular strength, and flexibility or posture.[710] When conducting trials most researchers focus on one or other type of exercise. Cardiovascular exercise may include jogging or swimming for example. Muscular strength could be sit-ups or weights.

---

[704] Boyes, 2015:181; Miller, 2009:226.
[705] Mondimore, 1999:227.
[706] Miller, 2009:226.
[707] Boyes, 2015:181.
[708] bipolarUK, 2018; NHS, 2016; Owen & Saunders, 2008:175.
[709] Khamba et al., 2011; NCCMH, 2006:21.
[710] Miller, 2009:101; North et al., 1990.

Flexibility or posture might be yoga or martial arts.

Over the past couple of decades "exercise on prescription" has become very popular in the UK.[711] GPs refer a patient to physiotherapy, hydrotherapy and exercise programmes for a number of injuries and illnesses, including bipolar depression.

Why is exercise important if you have BPII?

There is definitely a strong relationship between feeling physically good and feeling mentally good.[712] This is especially true when you consider the effects of exercise and good health on the body and brain.

Certainly the most significant mental health benefit for we with BPII is exercise's effect on depression. Multiple studies over the last few decades have explored the impact of exercise on unipolar and bipolar depressed patients. As a result of the numerous similar findings 'the mood-enhancing effect of exercise is [now] irrefutable'.[713] Most of the research in this area supports the conclusion that exercise has antidepressant qualities and can even completely relieve mild to moderate depression.[714] Some studies even suggest that exercise may be as efficient as antidepressant medications[715] or psychotherapy.[716] So if you are feeling depressed then a little exercise each day may genuinely help, even if it's just a 20 minute walk outside.[717]

---

[711] Lawlor & Hopker, 2001.

[712] Miller, 2009:100; Glenister, 1996.

[713] White, 2014:91.

[714] Woodridge, 2016:231; Boyes, 2015:167; White, 2014:119; Roberts et al., 2013:97; Eriksson & Gard, 2011; Marohn, 2011:51; NCCMH, 2006:390; Brown & Gerbarg, 2005; Lawlor & Hopker, 2001; Craft & Landers, 1998; Byrne & Byrne, 1993; LaFontaine, 1992; North et al., 1990.

[715] Eriksson & Gard, 2011.

[716] LaFontaine, 1992.

[717] Haycock, 2010:97; Wilkinson, 1999:37.

Another benefit of exercise important to those of us with BPII is its anxiolytic (anti-anxiety) effect. Again, an abundance of research supports the conclusion that exercise can reduce or even alleviate anxiety.[718]

Exercise has a preventative quality against the development of stress[719] and, as we know, stress can be a major factor in the triggering of bipolar mood episodes.

Another important benefit is that physical activity tires you out and relaxes you, meaning it is easier to get a restful night's sleep.[720]

Other positives include: counteracting weight gain caused as a meds side effect,[721] improved focus and concentration,[722] stimulation of the appetite,[723] reduction of hyperactivity and irritability,[724] enhancement of your metabolism[725] and increase in energy levels.[726] Also exercise obviously has positive physical health benefits in making us fitter and so less prone to fall ill.

In terms of exercise's effect on hypomania, there has been no clear research that I could find as yet. It is in my experience that exercise helps alleviate excess energy experienced during hypomania, but no trials yet corroborate this. It is possible that exercise may be helpful to people experiencing hypomania in this way, and prove a suitable distraction from racing thoughts. However it is just as possible that for some, exercise may further arouse the body creating more

---

[718] Boyes, 2015:167; Marohn, 2011:51; Brown & Gerbarg, 2005; Byrne & Byrne, 1993; LaFontaine, 1992; North et al., 1990.
[719] Marohn, 2011:51; Miller, 2009:35; Guyol, 2006:180; Brown & Gerbarg, 2005; Wilkinson, 1999:37; North et al., 1990.
[720] White, 2014:119; Marohn, 2011:51; Fieve, 2006:108; Brown & Gerbarg, 2005; Wilkinson, 1999:37; North et al., 1990.
[721] Hall-Flavin, 2012.
[722] Wooldridge, 2016:231; White, 2014:119; Brown & Gerbarg, 2005.
[723] Wilkinson, 1999:37.
[724] Marohn, 2011:51.
[725] Guyol, 2006:180.
[726] Guyol, 2006:180.

elation and greater energy levels, exacerbating hypomanic symptoms.[727]

Regardless of the positive effects of exercise on those of us with BPII, exercise 'should not replace standard treatment'.[728] Exercise is an excellent adjunct therapy and a sound self-management technique, particularly given that we with BPII are at greater risk for any number of fitness-related medical problems[729] and a lack of exercise can 'contribute to bipolar'.[730] In a study of people with psychiatric illnesses, it was found that people with bipolar were most likely to have gained more than ten pounds in the last six months, least likely to have been asked by their GP about their activity levels, and very likely to self-report 'poor exercise habits, including infrequent walking ... or strength exercises'.[731] So exercising should be a priority for people with BPII.

How does exercise work?

There are several theories why exercise has the effects on mood that it does, in reducing depression and anxiety. Here is a brief explanation of each:

- Cognitive Behavioural: basically, this theory follows the CBT model that changes in behaviour can lead to changes in thinking and mood. Taking part in regular exercise makes us feel good about ourselves because exercise is seen as a virtue, and this lifts our mood.[732]
- Social: the interpersonal connections of some exercise, such as team sports or jogging groups, increases our social

---

[727] NCCMH, 2006:390.
[728] Lawlor & Hopker, 2001.
[729] Roberts et al., 2013:96.
[730] Marohn, 2011:27.
[731] Kilbourne et al., 2007.
[732] Lawlor & Hopker, 2001; North et al., 1990.

contact, brings the attention of others, and helps us develop our communication skills.[733]
- Distraction: when we exercise we tend to focus purely on what we are doing, it is like a kind of mindfulness. It keeps us concentrating on one activity and the sensations associated with it, allowing us time out from our psychological burden.[734]
- Cardiovascular fitness: this theory is based on the concept that getting physically fitter automatically has a positive impact on our mental health.[735] Though this theory has been refuted because the positive effects of exercise seem to start from the very first session.[736]
- Amine hypothesis: there is a lot of evidence to support that exercise helps increase the concentration and enhance the activity of the neurotransmitters serotonin, norepinephrine and dopamine, all of which make us feel good.[737]
- Endorphins: exercise also releases feel-good hormones called endorphins, 'natural opiates' which also relieve pain.[738]
- Mastery: if we undertake an exercise which requires the development of skills, such as tennis, then mastery of those skills may increase our self-confidence and self-worth.[739]

Myself and most researchers agree that the causes for the mood-enhancing effects of exercise are a combination of the above.

---

[733] NCCMH, 2006:385; Lawlor & Hopker, 2001; North et al., 1990.
[734] Roberts et al., 2013:96; NCCMH, 2006:385; Lawlor & Hopker, 2001; North et al., 1990.
[735] Miller, 2009:92; North et al., 1990
[736] LaFontaine, 1992; North et al., 1990.
[737] Miller, 2009:37; Guyol, 2006:180; NCCMH, 2006:385; Lawlor & Hopker, 2001; North et al., 1990.
[738] Miller, 2009:100; Owen & Saunders, 2008:182; NCCMH, 2006:385; Lawlor & Hopker, 2001; North et al., 1990.
[739] NCCMH, 2006:385.

What types of activities count as exercise?

The most basic explanation is that any activity which either raises your pulse and breathing rate, or improves muscle tone and strength counts as exercise. 'This might amount to no more than a pleasant, brisk 20-minute walk'.[740] 'Walking is exercise'[741] and 'every step you take helps keep your mood stable and your heart and lungs happy'.[742] Yoga is exercise.[743] Riding a bike, swimming and jogging are all moderate intensity exercises.[744] Tennis, football, cricket and basketball are all moderate intensity sports.

The tricks are to, a) pick a 'physical activity level that's right for you',[745] b) plan activities that you enjoy,[746] and c) add in some variety.[747] If your current fitness level is low and you are prone to rumination then jogging may not be for you, try aquarobics or pilates instead. If you are already in good shape, then perhaps start jogging, join a gym and sign up to the local rugby team, as variety helps you stay motivated and wanting to exercise. If you struggle with motivation maybe get a friend to join you, or hire a personal trainer. If you find you don't have the time, money or inclination, start with simple things like parking your car at the far end of the parking lot, or walking to the second closest bus stop rather than the nearest. Do some stretches first thing in the morning (it'll help wake you up and is a really healthy way to start the day).

Whatever you do, pick something enjoyable and within your capabilities: push yourself, but not to the point where you hurt, for example don't start your jogging programme by immediately trying

---

[740] Wilkinson, 1999:37.
[741] Haycock, 2010:97.
[742] White, 2014:102.
[743] Owen & Saunders, 2008:188; Guyol, 2006:180-181; Brown & Gerbarg, 2005.
[744] White, 2014:102-103.
[745] Boyes, 2015:169.
[746] NHS, 2016.
[747] Miller, 2009:102.

to train for your local half-marathon, just tire yourself out for twenty minutes then come home gently.

Diet
Healthy body leads to healthy mind

A good base level of nutrition is essential for everyone to maintain 'optimal brain functioning and mood regulation'.[748] No matter whether or not you have BP, healthy diet and optimal nutrient levels are needed for us to function at our best. There is a vast array of evidence that a healthy diet is integral to a healthy mood.[749]

Good diet, good for BP:

Unfortunately, nutritional 'deficiencies and imbalances are a common feature of bipolar disorder';[750] in many cases people with BP 'self-report suboptimal eating behaviours'[751] which lead to reduced energy levels,[752] an inability to produce enough neurotransmitters[753] and, subsequently, can lead to depression[754] or other 'adverse neuropsychiatric effects'.[755]

What is a healthy diet for bipolar?

The NHS suggests that eating well and improving diet is a key element of bipolar management.[756] This is in part because obesity is a common problem for those of us with bipolar[757] as well as the reasons already given.

---

[748] White, 2014:63.
[749] Miller, 2009:95.
[750] Marohn, 2011:37.
[751] Kilbourne et al., 2007.
[752] Miller, 2009:92-93.
[753] Marohn, 2011:40.
[754] NCCMH, 2006:21.
[755] Freeman et al., 2006.
[756] NHS, 2016.
[757] Wildes et al., 2006.

Much of what constitutes a healthy diet for someone with BPII is similar to recommendations for all people, like:[758]

- Eat more fruits, vegetables and whole grains. Fruits and vegetables contain vital vitamins, like the B-complex vitamins which help keep depression at bay. Whole grains are a good source of fibre, very important as many BP meds can cause constipation.
- Switch to low-fat dairy products. A lot of BP meds cause weight gain, so reducing fats in our diets is never a bad thing.
- Minimise your intake of solid fats. Again, anything that helps us keep the weight off is good.
- Drink plenty of water. If you take lithium it is especially important to maintain a regular fluid intake to reduce the risk of toxicity. Some BP meds cause headaches and a good amount of water intake helps with this tremendously.

There are some ideas which may be particular to a BPII diet, such as avoiding or reducing caffeine.[759] Caffeine is a stimulant and may contribute to poor sleep and possibly even the development of hypomania. It is best to cut down on your caffeine levels, but if you simply enjoy your coffee, tea and cola too much, just avoid drinking them for a few hours before bedtime to help ensure a good night's sleep, because we know poor sleep can precipitate mood episodes.

Making sure you have a diet rich in B-vitamins helps to hold back depression because B_6 boosts serotonergic neurotransmission[760] and B_{12} and folate help avoid 'adverse neuropsychiatric effects'.[761] Foods that are rich in B-vitamins include: pork, ham, dark green leafy vegetables, whole grains, lentils, nuts, eggs and bananas.

---

[758] White, 2014:79-80.
[759] bipolarUK, 2018; White, 2014:76.
[760] Shabbir et al., 2013.
[761] Freeman et al., 2006.

Another nutrient, which is important to the production of serotonin, is tryptophan.[762] Some foods high in tryptophan include: oats, cheese, eggs, dark chocolate, milk, fish, sunflower seeds and quinoa.

As already noted, another key nutrient for positive bipolar management is omega-3. Omega-3 has protective qualities against mood disorders[763] and incurs other health benefits. The main food high in omega-3 is fish,[764] but it is better to eat ocean fish rather than farmed fish because it is eating algae that causes fish to be high in omega-3.[765] Omega-3 deficiency has even been suggested as being part of the cause of the emergence of bipolar disorder.[766]

Another product to avoid, or at least reduce, is alcohol as it has been shown to influence mood.[767] Alcohol is a depressant, ergo it can cause depressive symptoms to arise. If you don't want to cut alcohol completely from your diet, it is still recommended that you drink infrequently and certainly that you avoid binge-drinking.

It is important to remember that while some advice makes it feel like we must have the perfect diet all the time,[768] it is absolutely necessary that you don't take this to the extreme; don't beat yourself up for having the occasional milkshake or junk food.[769] And '[don't] move too quickly in your campaign for diet reform; only change a couple of products at a time, and add new foods rather than just cutting out those that you currently eat and are bad for you'.[770] Just try to eat a 'balanced' diet.[771]

---

[762] Shabbir et al., 2013.
[763] Freeman et al., 2006.
[764] NCCMH, 2006:377.
[765] McManamy, 2006:288.
[766] Marohn, 2011:37.
[767] White, 2014:76; Miller, 2009:99.
[768] Marohn, 2011:55; Miller, 2009:96.
[769] Haycock, 2010:96.
[770] Wilkinson, 1999:36-37.

Support Networks

What is a support network?

A support network is the group of people who help you to manage and cope with your bipolar. They are the people who offer you support, help, treatment and encouragement over the course of your bipolar journey, both when you are sick and when you are stable.

Who is in a support network?

There may be lots of different types of people in your support network, but they generally boil down to two groups: the professionals involved in your care and the people who help you on a day-to-day basis with managing your bipolar and life in general.

The first group, the professionals, may include your GP, psychiatrist, psychologist/psychotherapist, care co-ordinator, CPN (Community Psychiatric Nurse), social worker and crisis support team or emergency services.

In the latter group are friends, family, employers and colleagues. You could also include your care co-ordinator, CPN or social worker in this group.

What are their roles?

- GPs: Your GP is your first port of call. They make initial referrals to mental health services and other healthcare professionals, prescribe and monitor maintenance medication and take physical tests such as blood pressure, blood tests and ECGs all relevant to BPII and the meds used to treat it.[772]

---

[771] Owen & Saunders, 2008:175.
[772] Owen & Saunders, 2008:106-107.

- Psychiatrists: Your psychiatrist's jobs are to diagnose, manage and prevent mental ill health.[773] They prescribe acute phase and initial maintenance medications and make referrals to psychotherapy. They are also in charge of involving a CPN or social worker in your care. And they can help you create an Advanced Directive.
- Psychologists: Your psychologist is a non-medical professional. They focus primarily on psychotherapies such as CBT or IPSRT.[774]
- Care co-ordinators: The role of the care co-ordinator is quite expansive. Your care co-ordinator is most likely to be a CPN or social worker. They focus on you as a whole person and practise prevention as much as treatment, they can call emergency meetings with your psychiatrist if necessary, they liaise between yourself and your healthcare providers, they look out for early warning signs of incipient mood episodes, they provide help in understanding the treatments available to you, they perform risk assessment and risk management, they promote healthy living and they speak with family and carers, among other duties.[775] Their main focus is to get to know you well as a patient and as a person.[776]
- Crisis support team: Hopefully you will never need a crisis support/crisis resolution team, but should you find yourself experiencing a mental health crisis you can call them anytime, 24/7. Whenever possible they will be with you within four hours, will carry out an emergency mental health assessment and, if necessary, will provide short term aid.[777]
- Emergency services: Again, hopefully you will never have to use the emergency services, but if you find yourself in a

---

[773] Owen & Saunders, 2008:108.
[774] Owen & Saunders, 2008:109.
[775] Hodges, 2012:52; Owen & Saunders, 2008:110-111.
[776] Owen & Saunders, 2008:110.
[777] Owen & Saunder, 2008:113.

position where you feel actively suicidal or have taken actions towards suicide or self-harm, either get yourself to A&E or call for an ambulance. You will see the on-call/duty psychiatrist or mental health team and you will also be given any physical treatment you require.
- Family and friends: Your loved ones offer invaluable support making it easier for you to cope with your life with bipolar disorder.[778] They can help recognise prodromes (early warning signs), provide practical and emotional support, and help with appointments, aiding both you and the healthcare professionals.[779]
- Employers and colleagues: Your employer in particular can provide vital support in the workplace in the form of reasonable adjustments and understanding in the face of bouts of sick leave due to bipolar episodes.

Long term work with healthcare professionals 'is absolutely essential for our mental health'[780] and 'in addition to psychotherapy and medication adherence, social support [is] a significant factor in extending periods of wellness'.[781]

Why are support networks important?

There are a significant number of reasons why your support network is important. Here follows a list compiled from my own experiences and extensive research:[782]

- Engaging with the "real world" helps keep depression at bay

---

[778] Roberts et al., 2013:155.
[779] Owen & Saunders, 2008:117.
[780] Todd, 2016:22.
[781] Roberts et al., 2013:155.
[782] bipolarUK, 2018; Boyes, 2015:169-171; White, 2014:121-128; Roberts et al., 2013:161; Jackel, 2010; Miller, 2009:109; Fieve, 2006:243-244; NCCMH, 2006:21; Mondimore, 1999:228 & 240; Wilkinson, 1999:52.

- Spending time with loved ones increases your happiness and psychological wellbeing
- The more people who are there to help spot prodromes, the better
- Providing support through stress and coping with triggers that arise
- Providing financial support and advice
- Helping with employment issues and engaging in reasonable adjustments
- Assessing when mood and behaviour changes are normal or when they are bipolar-related
- Attending medical appointments with you
- Reminding you to take your meds
- Reminding you to do your psychotherapy or self-help exercises
- Meditating with you
- Exercising with you
- Sharing your healthier diet with you
- Helping you write an Advanced Directive
- Checking in with you on a regular basis
- Assisting with chores and childcare
- Making plans together to socialise
- Developing a maintenance/self-management programme with you
- Helping you to feel accepted
- Causing you to be more resilient against problems and set backs
- Keeping you accountable for your behaviour
- Stopping you from feeling isolated and lonely
- Understanding and encouraging you
- Aiding in resistance against poor physical health
- Creating contact with others, socialising
- Comforting us when we are in despair
- Reining us in when we are getting too high.

So, you see the list of reasons why support networks are important is quite long, and I would not even venture to assume that this list is exhaustive.

Support groups:

Support groups are places where people with similar problems meet together to share stories, support each other and combat loneliness. Groups like Alcoholics Anonymous are support groups.

Many people with bipolar disorder, and those with other mental health conditions, 'say that their most effective therapy – the kind that helps them move past their illness and on with their lives – comes from attending a support group'.[783]

In my opinion, the most important function of support groups is the development of the feeling that you are not alone, that you are not "different".[784]

Other key aspects of attending a support group are:[785]

- Providing information on prodromes (early warning signs and symptoms)
- Discussing medications and side effects
- Supporting each other in times of crisis
- Offering each other encouragement
- Sharing stories that might help others
- Making friends
- Providing helpful suggestions for tackling problems
- Having a safe place to air frustrations
- Developing greater acceptance of the illness

---

[783] Duke & Hochman, 1993:179.
[784] Haycock, 2010:96; Miller, 2009:240; McManamy, 2006:179; Mondimore, 1999:229; Wilkinson, 1999:70; Duke & Hochman, 1993:179.
[785] Roberts et al., 2013:163-164; Haycock, 2010:96; Miller, 2009:240; Fieve, 2006:244; McManamy, 2006:179; NCCMH, 2006:11; Mondimore, 1999:229; Wilkinson, 1999:54 & 70; Duke & Hochman, 1993:179.

- Listening to guest speakers
- Reducing stress and negative feelings
- Swapping coping strategies.

What to work out when constructing your support network:

The first thing to decide is what types of help you may need from your support network. It may help to more generally consider what types of assistance someone with any chronic illness might need.[786] Would you benefit from emotional support, such as help coming to terms with your diagnosis? Would you benefit from social support, such as company when exercising? Would you benefit from informational support, such as help understanding your medication regime? Would you benefit from practical support, such as assistance with groceries shopping?

Next, decide who you need these varying types of support from.[787] Don't just assume, actually have conversations with the relevant people and be realistic: your family may be willing and able to help with chores, but not your care co-ordinator. Conversely, your care co-ordinator should be able to help explain treatment options, but family members are unlikely to have the requisite knowledge. It is important to know who to call on.[788]

Telling People You Have Bipolar

There are lots of types of people we come across in life. Those people play different roles, from partners to employers to children. And there are lots of reasons why you might want or need to tell people you have bipolar disorder.

Who are we talking about?

In the context of informing people that we have bipolar, I think

---

[786] Fieve, 2006:242-243.
[787] Roberts et al., 2013:162.
[788] Mondimore, 1999:235-236.

people are split into three groups: people who need to know that we have bipolar disorder, people we want to know we have bipolar disorder, and people who we don't want to and do not need to know we have bipolar disorder. You are of course welcome to disagree; you may wish to take a different perspective on the world.

In my mind, people who need to know we have bipolar are: any health care professionals who treat us (for anything, not just our mental health), immediate family (those you live with), partners, our children (no matter what age they are), and employers. It is important for these people to know for varying reasons. Health care professionals need to know what treatments and medications you are receiving in order to not contradict your bipolar management programme. Employers need to know so they can put into place safe-guards in case you get ill and know that you may need either extra assistance or time off work periodically. And family, partners and children need to know as they spend the most time with us and are most likely to be affected by our bipolar mood states.

People we may want to know are friends and co-workers. Again this is because we spend a lot of time with these people. They may notice our erratic behaviours and mood swings; I think it is helpful for them to know there is a reason for this.

People we may not want to know, and who probably don't need to know are distant family and strangers. You may not want these people asking a lot of questions or butting into your business.

Personally, I tell all and sundry because I want to promote the positive public profile of bipolar disorder, and people only learn by asking questions. But it is perfectly understandable if there are groups of people you don't want to know.

When do we tell them?

Depending on who, there are different times you might want to tell people. There are no hard and fast rules, these are only my opinion.

Employers should be told once you've signed the contract. You are not obliged to tell people on your application, though I choose to do so. However, if you think your bipolar would have a dramatic impact on your ability to do a certain job, don't apply. But once you are in a position, you cannot be fired for disclosing that you have a bipolar diagnosis. The safest way I've found is to discuss your condition with the HR manager or directly with your boss, and give them some information sheets freely available from the Bipolar UK website.

When it comes to health professionals, just tell them as soon as it is convenient or when they ask what meds you're on or if you have any other health conditions.

With romantic partners the line is pretty fuzzy. I personally would tell someone on the second or third date, others might wait until it's clear the relationship is going somewhere. One thing is for sure, tell them before you move in together or combine any finances. Prospective partners really should know, again it's worth pointing out there are information sheets on the Bipolar UK website and there are a range of books out there targeted specifically at people with a bipolar loved one.

I think family should be told as soon as you are comfortable with your diagnosis, or sooner if you are a little confused because they can help you work things out.

When it comes to children I think bipolar disorder should be a common household topic from as soon as they can grasp a conversation. At a very young age children know when something is wrong. If they have a name for why Mummy can't get out of bed today or Daddy has a short fuse, it can really help them come to terms with the environment they live in. Keeping it quiet and trying to keep it hidden does no one any favours.

I think telling people is important. It helps you feel less burdened and less secretive, and it helps them to understand, be less judgemental and more forgiving. All in all, people knowing is good.

If people take it badly

In most cases if someone reacts badly to the news that you have bipolar it's because they don't know enough about it. If you can, encourage them to read the Bipolar UK info sheets. If not, you may have to leave them to it and hope they come around. If they begin to treat you negatively because you have bipolar, you may need to cut that person from your life.

If a co-worker reacts badly or begins to treat you differently, you should tell your boss or HR manager. They should talk to the person on your behalf or mediate any unpleasantness.

If you're boss reacts negatively or begins to treat you badly, you can call on your union rep or speak to someone at Mind, the Citizen's Advice Bureau or Bipolar UK for advice.

Hopefully these will not happen to you, but if it does seek the help and support of a friend and/or the appropriate professionals. It is still good that these people know now. At least you know where they stand and how they feel, so you can act accordingly.

How do we tell people?

I find with all these people, and I reckon everyone else really, just telling them and answering any questions they have is the best way to go about it. People are less scared of something if they know a little about it.

Again, there are no hard and fast rules, but here are some tips I've gathered over the years through experience and research:[789]

- Calm yourself down: It is normal to feel anxious when disclosing that you have a chronic condition,[790] but it is important to at least appear calm when having these conversations. If you can't calm yourself with some preparation and breathing exercises, remember to "fake it till you make it".
- Start with the people closest to you: These are the people who are most likely to have helped you in the past and who love you. They are the people most likely to be supportive and want to help.[791]
- Be well educated about your illness: You want to be able to explain fully and clearly what bipolar disorder is and how it affects not only you, but the person to whom you are disclosing your diagnosis.
- Find a suitable situation for the conversation: Make sure you pick a place with few distractions and an occasion when there is no definite time limit. You want to give this conversation the attention it deserves.
- Apologise if necessary: You may have in the past affected someone with your bipolar behaviours, so you may want to apologise for any grievance or upset you believe you may have caused.
- Be prepared to answer questions: There is still a lot of stigma surrounding mental health,[792] so you may have to answer some quite difficult questions about BP. Other questions may be very straightforward. You have to be prepared to answer both emotionally and knowledgably.
- Be honest: Don't play up your bipolar, but also don't play it down. The people you are telling need to know the truth about bipolar, warts and all.

---

[789] White, 2014:138-140; Roberts et al., 2013:158; Haycock, 2010:117.
[790] White, 2014:131.
[791] White, 2014:130; Mondimore, 1999:228.
[792] Paquette, 2016; Owen & Saunders, 2008:218.

- Offer further resources: For those close to you, books for the loved ones of people with bipolar disorder exist. There are also plenty of online resources for friends, health professionals and employers.

Friends with Mental Health Disorders
Shared experience

I have noticed a common trait in people with or who in the past have experienced mental health issues: we surround ourselves with a lot of other people with or who have had mental illness; and not just the disorder that you've got. I have had friends with bipolar, depression, borderline personality disorder (BPD), anxiety, PTSD and eating disorders. We are like homing beacons for each other; the shared experiences and feelings can make us fast friends. That's not to say that I like everyone I've met with a mental health disorder, I don't, but an awful lot of my friends have some sort of mental health issue. From talking to lots of people, this seems to be fairly normal for us. Generally having friends who understand and share your experiences is a good thing, but it can present problems.

The good things

There are such great positives to having friends who also have mental health conditions.

For one, it's just nice to know we're not alone. Even if none of your friends specifically have BPII, knowing there are other people struggling with their mental health makes you feel a little less lonely.

You can share; it's really supporting and supportive to be able to share your stories and experiences with other people who may have similar stories and experiences.

There is no judgement; if you've done something ill-advised on account of your mental health, like self-harm, it is unlikely that your friends with mental health issues are going to be judgemental or hold it against you.

Empathy; not only do your friends care for you, these friends can actually empathise as well. And you can empathise with them, which feels good.

Mutual support; you get to help look out for each other, which is a healthy positive social interaction.

Anxiety-lite socialising: you know that you are safer around your friends, and safer still when those friends have similar difficulties to you. You are subsequently less likely to feel anxious in the first place. But should you become anxious these friends tend to be more understanding and will either give you assistance or space, depending on which you need.

The problems

If you have a friend who dips in and out of depression or experiences fluctuating anxiety or has panic attacks, then you have a friend who needs varying types and levels of support at different times. You will want to be there for them. It's only fair, they will have been there for you and will probably do it again. And sometimes helping a friend is good for us; on a physical level as well as emotional. But sometimes it's bad for us.

How?

1. If you're like me you take on emotional baggage. So say, your friend with PTSD needs support and tells you all about their trauma, you may go home and ruminate on it until it makes you so upset you get stuck in a loop.
2. It may make you feel guilty. Such as, "so-and-so has it way worse than me, what do I have to get ill over?" You can

end up pondering whether you have the <u>right</u> to be poorly. This is bad as it leads to negative cyclic thinking and unpleasant emotions.
3. It may resonate too much. What your friend is going through may be too similar to a bad experience you have had yourself. This can merge your past with their present and make you not only useless to them, but stuck in a vicious mental cycle of reliving your own unpleasant experience.
4. This is a biggy: It may trigger you. If you're helping a friend in a difficult situation or a dangerous mood state, you may find your own negative thought patterns and emotions are triggered and you end up spiralling into a similar situation or mood state.

So what do you do?

Well first you have to decide if you are well enough to cope and actually help. If you're too high or too low you put yourself at greater risk of the problems described above and may actually make things worse for your friend too. If you are not fit to deal with this situation, say so and, if you can, tag someone else in. Say, "I'm sorry, but at the moment I am not equipped to help you. Who else can I call who might be able to help?" You are doing the right thing for yourself and actually for your friend too. You are being more helpful than if you put yourself into a situation you couldn't safely handle.

If you are fit enough, you go. But you may still find it turns out to be bad for you after. If that happens, you need to recharge and calm down. I recommend doing your 'wasting time with a purpose' activity (see the section for more information). And if that doesn't work, talk to someone in your own support network (see section for more information). You are allowed to ask for help too.

Taking care of yourself

When I say being 'selfish' I mean more looking after yourself before helping others to the detriment of your own mental health and well-being.

Sometimes being selfish means making a couple of tough decisions. It often means getting more advanced help than you can offer.

- Do you need to call the CPN, psychiatrist etc. for this person? Explain that you think it would be best and try to get them to make the phone call for themselves, if not you may need to make a phone call on their behalf. Calling the right mental health worker: there is no hard and fast rule, but remember this can apply to calling for yourself not just on the behalf of a friend.
    - If it's definitely a medication issue like horrible, unbearable side effects, you need to call the psychiatrist's clinic and ask for an emergency appointment. You/your friend should not stop taking the medication unless instructed by a psychiatrist or GP.
    - If it's about emergency support in a crisis, call the Home Management/Crisis Team; most clinics either have one or work with one.
    - If it's about psychological or practical care then call the CPN or social worker and ask to speak to the duty worker.
    - There may be others assigned to a person's mental health team, they will know who.
- Do you need to call an ambulance? If a person is at immediate risk of or has already made actions towards self-harm or suicide, call an ambulance. They need to be in a place of safety as soon as possible and that can only be assured by calling an ambulance. It is also the best way to

get emergency treatment after any self-harm or suicide attempts.
- Do you need to call the police? If a person is a risk to the safety of others then you must call the police. Be sure to explain the situation and person's diagnosis clearly, this will help the police know how to handle the situation and whether the person needs to be held under the Mental Health Act. You cannot allow someone to be a danger to other people, if that means spending a night in detention it is better than risking the safety of yourself or others.
- Do you need to end this relationship? Some relationships become toxic. You may find that you are always helping someone and always feel awful or drained afterwards. You may find you dread seeing someone. If you can bring yourself to, talk to them and explain your problems; this may lead to a healthier relationship. If not, break it off. You have to look after yourself first.

Mindfulness

In Western culture mindfulness is still a relatively new concept, but it has its roots in Eastern spiritual practices[793] possibly going back a thousand years or more. Mindfulness is a peaceful, relaxing type of meditation and self-awareness. The best short description I've found is:

mindfulness is "paying attention in a particular way: on purpose, in the present moment, and non-judgmentally"[794]

To break it down:

'in a particular way': This is a twofold process; first it is paying attention to your surroundings, what you can feel, see, hear, taste and smell. Secondly, it is paying attention to yourself, your body

---

[793] Kabat-Zinn, 1990 in Roberts et al., 2013:92.
[794] Kabat-Zinn, 1994, 4 in Roberts et al., 2013:92.

sensations, thoughts and emotions. The first part is much easier than the second, so when learning mindfulness you usually start with exercises that focus on your surroundings or on imagery, and then you move to exercises where you focus on yourself.

'on purpose': this means it is a deliberate act. Sometimes we are, most of us, accidentally mindful of our surroundings and ourselves. We may take a stroll in the countryside and find we are listening to the birds, touching the trees and enjoying the warmth of the sun on our face. Shifting this to deliberately focusing on these things, turns the process into a form of mindfulness. Taking a few deep breaths to calm ourselves down is accidental mindfulness. Shifting to consciously acknowledge the feeling of the air as it passes through your nose, throat and down into your lungs, becomes mindful meditation.

'in the present moment': this is where things start to get difficult. It is relatively easy to focus on the surroundings we find ourselves in, but when it comes to paying attention to our own thoughts and emotions we often end up thinking about the past or the future. When this happens we must gently bring ourselves back to the present.[795] It is a normal part of mindfulness, it will happen a fair bit, don't worry about it, just come back to how you're feeling now, what you are thinking about yourself right now.

'non-judgmentally': this is hands-down the most difficult part of mindfulness. You may notice that you are feeling angry, for example, and then start thinking about how you are weak or unstable for being angry. In mindfulness you are instead supposed to simply acknowledge your anger, accept that it is a present emotion, not a reflection upon yourself, and then move on. Move on to the next emotion or thought, or return to your body sensations or surroundings for a while because it is easier to be

---

[795] Boyes, 2015:90.

neutral about those things.

Why practise mindfulness?

There is an accumulating body of evidence gathered to show that mindfulness has a positive impact on the mental health of those with bipolar.[796] It is particularly helpful in reducing symptoms of anxiety.[797]

Mindfulness practice has been shown to have a number of positive effects:[798]

- building emotional awareness[799]
- reducing unhealthy coping mechanisms
- gaining better control of your thoughts
- improving memory and concentration
- creating more positive emotions
- relaxing.

Mindfulness also helps to combat rumination (over-thinking about the past or future) which is a common symptom of depression and has been shown to prolong depressive episodes.[800]

Mindfulness exercises

Mindfulness exercises can start as very small practices and become much longer, more complex meditations. To begin with it may be as simple as focusing on the sensations of one big, deep breath before you get out of bed in the morning.[801] It may be three minutes of sitting quietly and observing your body sensations.[802] It may be an

---

[796] Perich et al., 2013; Deckersbach et al., 2012.
[797] Boyes, 2015:89.
[798] Van Dijk, 2009 in Roberts et al., 2013:94-95.
[799] Miller, 2009:30.
[800] Nolen-Hoeksema, 1991.
[801] Boyes, 2015:168.
[802] Boyes, 2015:89.

imagery technique.

I am going to describe for you two techniques I have found useful and calming.

First is a relatively short, straight-forward exercise I call 'coffee mindfulness':

-   Make your favourite hot drink; coffee, chai, hot chocolate, whatever makes you feel happy. Make it in a mug or cup, not a flask. Make it just cool enough to drink.
-   Take it somewhere you can sit down and have both hands on the cup. (I go outside and sit at the garden table.)
-   Plonk your bum down and notice your breathing. Slow it down a little and count to ten.
-   Then look at your drink and loosely wrap both of your hands around the mug.
-   Now observe your drink.
-   Start with the vessel: what colour is it? Is there a picture or pattern? Is it small or large? Describe the cup in your mind. How does it feel in your hands? Acknowledge the warmth in your palms versus the cold handle against your knuckles. Explain as many details as possible.
-   Now move to the drink itself. What colour is it? Be precise. How does it smell? Is there steam rising from it? Imagine how it is going to taste and how that will make you feel.
-   Bring the cup to your face; is the smell stronger? Can you feel the warmth against your face?
-   Take a sip and roll it around your mouth. How does it taste? Are there subtle flavours you haven't noticed before? Does it remind you of anything?
-   Swallow it and feel the warmth going down your throat. Imagine it heating up your whole body.
-   Drink some more. Observe how you react; did you sigh? Did you make an 'mmm' noise?

- Bring yourself back to the cup. Describe it again.
- Then count down from ten slowly, breathing in time with your counting.
- Bring yourself back to your surroundings.

Second is a more elongated imagery technique. Here's how it goes, step by step:

- Make yourself comfortable; sit in a comfy chair or lie on your bed.
- Close your eyes and breathe naturally, don't change it in any way.
- In your "mind's eye", imagination or whatever you want to call it picture a door, any door you like; sliding, glass, wooden, electric, whatever (just not a car door, else this won't work).
- Open the door and see in front of you an escalator going down.
- Step on the escalator and notice there are numbers on the walls in regular increments, ten to one. Count with them as you go down, ten to one.
- When you reach the number one at the bottom, step off the escalator. Stop and once again take note of your natural breathing.
- There's a plain wooden door in front of you, like the doors to rooms in an old house.
- Open the door and step through.
- See all around you a light and airy woodland. The golden sun is dappling through the trees. A light breeze rustles the leaves and your clothes. Soft moss and lush grass are underfoot. Small granite boulders are dotted around.
- You see a gentle winding path leading through the trees; follow it slowly.
- At the end of the trail you come to a glade. The blue sky above has cotton-ball clouds skittering by. In the centre of the

clearing is a pool; the water is still and shining like a mirror, clear down to the rocks and sand at the bottom of the basin. Around the edge are tufts of grass, reeds and a small stone slab covered in spongey dry moss.

- Go sit on the stone, take off your shoes and socks and dip your feet in the cool water.
- Just sit a while and observe what is around you. If your mind wanders, don't worry minds do that, just bring yourself back to the rough bark of the trees, the warmth of the sun on your skin, the silky water between your toes.
- When you're ready, go back to the door.
- Register your breathing; don't change it in any way.
- Step back through the door onto the escalator and this time count up with the numbers from one to ten.
- At the top step back through your door and then slowly open your eyes.
- Slowly come back to the room around you.
- Notice your breathing again, and that's the end of the exercise.

I hope you find these exercises helpful, I know they helped me.

Writing to Keep Us on Track

When you have BPII, there are a lot of reasons to write things down, many of which can help you to stay healthy and monitor yourself. The three main categories I recommend are journals, mood trackers and schedules. Each of these helps us in slightly different ways, but they are all useful.

Journals:

A journal, or a diary, is a book (or even a computer document or blog) where you write down the events of the day, your thoughts and feelings and anything else that's important to you. You may also write in your self-help book or psychotherapy exercises like I do. A lot of researchers have supported the theory that writing in a journal is helpful to our mental health.[803] Journals help us to work through our thoughts and emotions in a more constructive and healthier way. Having it written down makes it more tangible and therefore simpler to address. If nothing else, it helps us to remember which things we want to talk to our Care Co-ordinator, psychiatrist or psychologist about.

Mood trackers:

A mood tracker, mood map or life map is essentially, in its most basic form, a chart of your mood from day-to-day. It may be as simple as a list in the back of your journal where you write the date and a number to rate your mood for the day (a common scale is 0-10 where 0 is suicidal and catatonic, 5 is stable and 10 is psychotic manic; if you have BPII you probably will only rarely even reach an 8). In its more comprehensive forms you may record your mood rating in the morning and the evening, how much you slept, how anxious and how irritable you were, medication changes and any major life events. In this way you keep track of triggers as well as basic mood ratings and other BP symptoms. Keeping a mood tracker is widely recommended.[804]

Schedules:

Keeping track of what you're doing and when is a really helpful way to keep your life in order and make sure that you're getting done everything you need to stay healthy. You can keep a dates diary, calendar or wallchart, whichever suits you. Make sure to write down any appointments you have, when you plan to exercise, when you plan to take a bath or do some meditation, when you're going

---

[803] White, 2014:9; Hodges, 2012:68; Kennard, 2011:25; Mondimore, 1999:227; Lepore, 1997.
[804] NIMH, 2018; White, 2014:8 & 29; Miller, 2009:239-240; Kennard, 2011:25; Miller, 2009:27; Fieve, 2006:232-235; NCCMH, 2006:22; Mondimore, 1999:227; Duke & Hochman, 1993:162.

to socialise, when you're going to do chores like the vacuuming and groceries shopping, and perhaps even a meal plan. It's easier to make sure you're sticking to all your healthy lifestyle habits if you keep a plan of when you're going to do each thing. Maybe you don't need to put your sleep/wake alarms down, because they should ideally be the same every day.

Creativity
Genius and insanity

In general terms, mental health conditions ("insanities") such as bipolar disorder, have long been associated with "genius":

- 'while not all individuals with Bipolar II are geniuses, I estimate that without some form of Bipolar II hypomania, there would be fewer geniuses!'[805]
- Madness in general 'has long been paired with genius in the arts'.[806]
- 'Many people have long shared [the] suspicion that genius and insanity are entwined'.[807]
- 'Human beings have speculated about the relationship between inspiration and insanity for centuries. Even pre-Grecian myths drew a connection between being mad and being singled out by the gods'.[808]

Creativity in the literature

In a lot of books about bipolar there is a section about creativity and I have found several articles on creativity as well. If you are particularly interested in the apparent connection between bipolar and creativity then I highly recommend a lot of work by Kay Redfield Jamison, in particular her book 'Touched with Fire'.

---

[805] Fieve, 2006:131.
[806] Marohn, 2011:12-13.
[807] Jamison, 1997.
[808] Duke & Hochman, 1993:214.

Many of the books draw a correlation between bipolar and the creative arts, especially during the hypomanic phase. Here are some of my findings:

- 'Hypomania can be a heightened, ebullient mood characterized by infatiguable energy, a flood of ideas, and – more often than is usually credited – profound accomplishment'.[809]
- People with bipolar have 'sharpened and unusually creative thinking'.[810]
- 'Scores' of poets, artists and composers have been 'similarly afflicted' with suspected bipolar.[811]
- 'Depression and mania may have a way of coaxing out the most noble and creative and visionary in us'.[812]
- Bipolar 'can sometimes enhance or otherwise contribute to creativity in some people'.[813]
- 'there is no doubt that bipolar disorder and creativity are linked'.[814]
- 'You may feel very creative and view the manic phase as a positive experience'.[815]
- 'The prevalence of bipolar disorder is simply much higher in groups of accomplished artists than in the general population'.[816]
- 'patients want to experience hypomania as it facilitates creativity, productivity at work and the possible achievement of goals'.[817]

Estimates, depending on who you're reading, put the percentage of

---

[809] Fieve, 2006:130.
[810] Jamison, 1993:103.
[811] Jamison, 1997.
[812] McManamy, 2006:83.
[813] Jamison, 1997.
[814] Hodges, 2012:22.
[815] NHS, 2016.
[816] Mondimore, 1999:213.
[817] NCCMH, 2006:201.

artists, writers and musicians/composers with bipolar disorder between 5% and 80%.[818] I'm willing to bet in that case that it's about 42.5% as that's about half way between the two. Back in 1921, even Emil Kraeplin 'commented on [bipolar's] connection with creativity'.[819]

The flip side

Because of the long list of people with bipolar disorder famous for art, acting, politics, music and business is quite extensive, it can be easy to romanticise bipolar disorder, and hypomania in particular. But bipolar 'is not a disease to be taken lightly. Nor is it one that should be wished for even by creative people'.[820]

And besides neither are all people with bipolar extraordinarily creative, nor are most artists prone to mood swings.[821] We are not all Van Goghs waiting for inspiration to strike; we cannot all be that creative. It is also unfair to give all the credit for our creativity to our bipolar, to do so is 'to admit that we are little more than mere puppets on a string'.[822]

What is creativity?

In my opinion creativity is about much more than being a world-class composer or Poet Laureate. It is also in the small things: if you write a blog, you are creative. If you do colouring books, you are creative. If you arrange your tea cupboard by the colour of the boxes, then you are creative. Creativity is about more than grand artistic pursuits. It may be knitting, doing nail art, writing a journal or keeping holiday scrap books. Just because we don't all paint great works of art and become famous, doesn't mean we don't

---

[818] Mondimore, 1999:211; Jamison, 1997; Duke & Hochman, 1993:216.
[819] Duke & Hochman, 1993:214.
[820] Duke & Hochman, 1993:221.
[821] Jamison, 1997.
[822] McManamy, 2006:83.

have a creative bone in our bodies.

Why is creativity important?

When we talk about positive healthy lifestyle for bipolar disorder, we often talk about scheduling in relaxation time. For a lot of people creative pursuits are relaxing. Whether it's doing cross stitch, learning a musical instrument or reorganising your book shelves by genre, these activities can be very calming.

On the other side of the coin, however, the thing a lot of the literature forgets to mention is the negative aspect of creativity: the frustration when things don't turn out as you hoped, the feelings of worthlessness you can develop if you're not very good at something you're trying out, the self-condemnation when you don't have the motivation to undertake your creative endeavours...

So, something really important to remember about creativity is that there is a time, a place and a mood for getting creative. It's important to know when to pursue creativity. If you're having trouble concentrating, it may be unwise to try starting that new crotchet pattern you found. If you have the meds side effect of tremors, perhaps you shouldn't tinker with your car engine or work with power tools. Instead try reorganising your kitchen or planning your next creative project.

And don't just rely on hypomania; remember we're only hypo 1% of the time. Use your depression too. That strength of emotion can drive creativity just as much as the flight of ideas from hypomania. And when we're depressed we also need more down-time. Take some time out every day to relax, and if you have the concentration and motivation, get creative. Don't forget, even dyeing your hair a funny colour is creative; there's a lot of scope.

Wasting Time with a Purpose

I don't really care who you are, everyone needs down time. Everyone's down-time is different, what is relaxing for one person is definitely not for someone else. And what some people do to chill, others may say is wasting time. I reckon that's okay. What's important is that you do something relaxing on a regular basis.[823]

I have found that even when stable, people with BPII (and people with many other mental health issues) need a little or a lot more down-time than healthy people. I know I do. But because I do I often berate myself for "wasting time". Some days I might need to use the whole day as down-time. Some days I don't need any; those are far fewer.

I think wasting time with a purpose is important to good mental health. Going to the gym or playing sports wastes time but releases endorphins and keeps you fit, so if that's your thing, do it. Doing puzzle books uses up your time, but keeps your brain focused and working hard. Even watching TV gives us an escape from our sometimes painful lives, this is good. Activities like knitting or fishing can be very relaxing.[824]

There is nothing wrong with wasting time as long as you're not just sat on the floor staring at a wall for four hours (I reckon I'm not the only one who's done that); that's not healthy. No matter what it is that you do, remind yourself why doing this is good for you, remember you are probably not just "wasting time".

---

[823] bipolarUK, 2018; Kennard, 2011:28; NCCMH, 2006:21.
[824] White, 2014:89.

Chapter Five:

My Musings

Wellness Language

It is really difficult when you have bipolar to cope with the way some people talk about mental health disorders. It is difficult sometimes to cope with how we talk about our own mental illness. How many times have a berated myself, "Stop it, you shouldn't be behaving like this; it's all in your head!"? How many times have I said, "I **am** bipolar"? I don't know... maybe every single day... still.

What I say to others

I've told plenty of people I have bipolar disorder, I have also told people I have a mental health issue (that goes down better because it's vaguer, and the more ambiguous the less scary). Some people I have simply told I don't cope well with stress, because you can't tell some people you have bipolar as that would automatically make you a madman and a danger to others. Unfortunately, we sometimes still have to be vague.

We don't know how to talk about mental health

The main reason people don't know how to talk about mental health is because we just don't talk about it, or at least as little as possible. It's changing, but it's still there. I received some lessons on mental health in secondary school, but I reckon it equated to fewer than ten hours across five years at school. It's a little better in most British schools these days. But how many adults do you reckon could explain the differences between bipolar and schizophrenia, or psychopathy and sociopathy, or even between OCD and being a 'clean-freak'? I bet you know a few because we surround ourselves with people who care to know the difference, but there aren't all that many out there yet. But that will change with education.

So, talking about mental (ill) health... How many times have you heard someone say, 'I'm/she's/he's so OCD'? So many times that you're not actually sure? Yeah, me too. I used to say it myself, before I started thinking about these things properly. Or when was the last time someone said, 'she was so psycho last week'? I very much doubt they were actually psychotic; did they see things that weren't there? Was Bugs Bunny telling them to steal all the carrots from the corner shop? Did they believe they could fly? No? Then they weren't "psycho". If someone has a bad day at work or is snappy, you say they were grouchy or angry or snippish, not psycho, it makes more sense too. Medical diagnoses are not everyday adjectives and I think everyone should be responsible for removing this function.

I think depressed is the most common one. Most people use depressed as a synonym for pretty sad or not really wanting to do much. For those of us who have been depressed, as in diagnosed with some kind of depressive episode levels of depressed, this sounds like an alright sort of day. I get frustrated when friends say, 'that was really depressing' when what they mean is, 'that was sad'. But depressed is common parlance. To say something is depressing just means it's sad or unfortunate or you don't want to think about it. As a result, when most people find something 'depressing' they try to put it out of their head and succeed quickly; people who are depressed cannot. For example, when the average neuroneutral person sees the Save the Children advert on TV they might think to themselves, 'that's really depressing' but by two adverts later that thought and any accompanying emotions have evaporated. Comparatively, when I am depressed, and I see that advert I burst into tears and then spend the next hour feeling guilty for being depressed when there are children out there without even somewhere to sleep. I feel guilty because I have food, water, clothes and a roof. My house hasn't been bombed, my country isn't war-torn, my parents are alive. I spend an hour hating and berating myself for being such a loathsome creature. An hour minimum. For me, the Save the Children advert is truly depressing, for a healthy person it is saddening.

Throw-away comments

These are things people 'just say'; they didn't think about it because they say this kind of thing all the time. These are things that a lot of people without mental health disorders might not think would upset, offend or trigger us. Of all the throw-away comments I've ever heard, the worst one is easy to pick: "I'd rather slit my wrists than..." You hear stuff like this all the time, and not just in social situations but at work too. It's just a saying, but the damage this phrase has inflicted upon me on several occasions is indescribable in many ways. The chain of emotional and psychological steps happens so fast it is hard to follow, but the point remains. Hyperbole is all well and good, but perhaps we need to start warding people away from such phrases. In this situation I choose, "there are a hundred other things I'd rather do right now".

But to be honest, even comments which really cannot be offensive can trigger some pretty nasty reactions in people with mental health problems. Again, this is not usually the intention of the user, but as a society we need to work on it. There are really two kinds of trigger comment: one causes a mood shift, the other causes an exasperation within a mood episode. We've seen the first group above. The second group is much more varied and has a lot to do with you as a person not just your mental health.

There are some exasperation comments which many of my friends with mental health issues have found to be particularly unhelpful when poorly. An example which I've discussed with several people, I have found makes every single one of them get up in arms: I had been ill already for a couple of weeks; rapid cycling dysphoric depression. I went to visit my folks. The next day I had a blocked nose, the next day I was sneezing and coughing. My mum said, "See now you're ill". Obviously, she was not making a reference to my bipolar, why would she? She was just commenting that because I was sneezing it was clear I now had a cold. I don't clearly remember a lot from those weeks, so it's quite possible she had mentioned my sniffles the day before and I had brushed them off as I often did.

That being said, regardless of what she meant or how she said it, my momentarily irate and depressive state meant that I simultaneously wanted to burst into tears and punch her square in the face. I somehow managed to get into the kitchen before I started shaking, part anger, part distress. Eventually my body opted for crying, possibly because I have spent well over a decade supressing any outward displays of anger; and anger itself really. When I'm well I simply cannot describe myself as ever being angry at other people.

But the point is, this completely innocuous remark from my mother (who by this point was working really hard at being empathetic to the point of ridiculousness), this one comment caused such a violent reaction in my bipolar inflamed brain that I spent the next hour crying and telling myself that she was right, I wasn't ill before having a cold. Did my mum say she thought I was ill before I started sneezing? No, said bipolar brain. Did she ever say that bipolar was less significant than a cold? No said logical brain. Did she ever say that bipolar was not an illness? No, in fact she often refers to it as '[my] illness'. But that didn't matter. My being acutely ill turned it all around in my head.

This does however link to my next language issue: vocabulary. Most pointedly, how we refer to mental health in general, how we refer to those with mental health issues and how we ask about it. My favourite terrible description of my bipolar was definitely it being called my 'affliction'; how old fashioned and demeaning. Affliction made it sound like a) it was contagious and b) I should be in an institution.

I already touched at the beginning of this section on the epic difference between 'am' and 'have'. All the time people use 'am' or 'is' to talk about people with mental health disorders. We talk about ourselves in terms of 'I am bipolar', I still do it all the time; but I'm not, I **have** bipolar. In fact, nowadays if I catch myself thinking or saying 'I am bipolar' I try to correct myself with the phrase, 'I have bipolar, I am not my bipolar. Bipolar is a part of me, but bipolar is not my defining feature'.

Next, what about when people ask about your Mental Health Disorder? I mean people who know you have one and want to ask how you are. 'So how have you been with the... y'know...' *wiggles fingers next to temple*. 'Oh, my bipolar?' she says as loudly as possible in the very crowded coffee shop to show it's okay, I'm not embarrassed. But it can be in private too.

Or when you apologise for something. Like my favourite: me, 'sorry for not really talking yesterday, I was having a low day; brain disengaged somewhat'. Person who doesn't have bipolar, 'it's okay, I know it was just your um... er... affliction.' WHAT? Are we in the 19th century? Am I damsel come down with the vapours? The Middle Ages and I've got a severe case of roaming demons in my head? NO! We know what it is, and yes, it's scary, but we don't omit the word cancer or stroke so don't miss out my legitimate medical diagnosis, it's bipolar, and it's not contagious. What's more, it signals that talking about it makes you uncomfortable, which makes me uncomfortable around you. So now I won't talk to you about it, which is probably great for you, but for me it ticks another person off the list of people I can trust and keep as part of my support network. One fewer in the compilation of people I could ask for help in the future.

How we talk to ourselves about our BPII

Now we come to your own head, tiny touch of CBT here so brace yourself. How do you talk to yourself in your head about your mental health and yourself in general? And is it healthy? Or helpful? Some of you will treat yourself with compassion and respect most of the time, but like me a lot of you won't most of the time. I know that in my own head I am quite damning and recriminating about my bipolar and quite unpleasant about myself. And speaking to other people with mental health disorders, this is really common. But it's difficult to overcome. For some people the concept that there's another way to think is confusing, or daunting.

For me this is sometimes the case. I am usually very self-critical. Obviously in some aspects of life this can be really helpful in the beginning. For example, in work self-evaluation is critical to improvement, but when it moves from useful evaluation to unfriendly self-criticism it is no longer healthy or helpful.

A touch of CBT

Here's one of the CBT tools I use on a regular basis. It's called cognitive restructuring. Basically, you notice you're thinking something negative about yourself or your mental health: my personal favourite being, "Eleanor, come on, it's all in your head, why do you have to be so stupid all the time?" The next step is to come up with a more realistic statement in response to counter the original negative thought. One way of doing this is to imagine what you would say to a friend if that thought was theirs. For my thought it'd be something like, 'It's not all in your head, you have a disorder that affects your whole being. You are not stupid; you're just in a funk. You need to take some time to relax and think about what to do next.' I have taken my original thought, changed the perspective on the first part and countered the second. This is cognitive restructuring. What I also like to do, if I'm alone, is to repeat aloud the counter statement a few times to fix it in my mind.

So, I still tell myself all the time things like 'get over it', 'it's just the bipolar talking' or 'I'm stupid', but when I remember, I restructure. And the more I do it, the more often I remember to do it. Keeping a notebook on me to jot things down when they pop into my head helps.

A touch of mindfulness

Of course, sometimes changing a particular thought is very difficult; sometimes the thought consumes your mind. Then you have to let the thought be, accept it's there, do nothing to it or with it, just let it exist. This is a step in mindfulness, not trying to make your thoughts do anything; just notice and accept. We've accidentally been doing it for years with positive thoughts, it's more difficult with the negative ones as they tend to cascade into a stream of other negative thoughts. But again, the more often you try, the more often it'll work. If you let your thought alone, it will pass; and you will realise that. You will notice its coming and going but it'll have no lasting effect on you. I thought this was utter rubbish when I was learning it. It took me years of thinking about it and talking to a BPI friend who finds mindfulness useful before I could get my head around it. See none of the books point out that we've been doing this with our positive and neutral thoughts for our whole lives.

All in all, the most important thing to remember when it comes to thinking negatively about yourself is: if you can't change it, don't dwell on it. Whether it's a slip of the metaphorical tongue thinking 'I am' rather than 'I have' or something far more sinister like 'I'm useless, it would be better if I were dead', it is only a thought and thoughts can be challenged or passed over. Maybe even say to yourself, "Thoughts can be challenged or passed over; they're only thoughts."

Bipolar Man's Best Friend: pets and mental illness

My family currently have two dogs, Seren and Bear. I love our dogs and I genuinely believe they love me back in their own simple way. We treat our dogs well, and they treat us well in return. I have a few bipolar friends with cats. I have a friend with recurrent depression who has a veritable menagerie. I have actually a lot of friends with various mental health issues who keep animals of some kind; furry, fishy, feathery and scaley. We all give lots of reasons why we have pets and why they are good for us. There are quite a few.

Why are pets good for us?

- They distract us:[825] Looking after and loving a pet gives us plenty to distract ourselves on a daily basis.
- Love: We love them unrelentingly and we know they love us back unconditionally even when we think no one could love us.[826]
- They are intuitive:[827] They know when we're sad; when I'm going through a depressive phase or having a bad day Seren follows me around. She is never more than a cuddle away unless she's asleep.
- Contact: physical contact with animals has been proven to release positive endorphins which make us feel better.
- They need us: We have to take care of them; feeding them means getting up in the morning, grooming them means we have to focus on a productive and pleasurable task, cleaning up after them helps us to feel grounded in the world, walking or playing with them keeps us active.[828]
- They are calming: Whether you are watching them swim round the aquarium or snuggled up with them on the sofa, you feel calmed by their presence.[829]
- They are company: Even if you live alone, you are never truly alone if you have a pet.[830]

---

[825] Miller, 2009:179.
[826] Forbes, 2015.
[827] Forbes, 2015; Miller, 2009:179.
[828] Miller, 2009:179.
[829] Forbes, 2015.
[830] Forbes, 2015.

- You can talk to them: your pets don't judge, they are just there, they listen because you're talking not because they have to. You can rant to them, confide in them and share your secrets and joys. They are just there listening to you.
- They cut stress levels & anxiety: spending time around animals, especially ones you can touch, has been proven to reduce stress and anxiety.[831]
- They keep us alive: Especially if you are the sole owner of your animals, even when you're suicidal you may worry what will happen to your animals if you die. It might be enough to stop you from committing suicide.

So pets I feel are an amazing part of the lives of many people with mental illness. Pets could even be part of your support network. I think pets are good for just about anyone, but I would recommend that if you have a mental health disorder (and you can afford it) you get a pet. They may just be another source of joy, but they may even save your life. Alternatively, you can "borrow" pets from your friends; take your mate's dog for a walk, have a cuddle with a guinea pig when you visit, watch the fish with them over a cup of tea; it helps. You could even cat-sit if your friend has to go away for some reason.

My Bipolar Idols

I have a lot of respect for people in many walks of life, but these are a few in the public eye for whom I have particular respect. My five bipolar idols are: Kay Redfield Jamison, Julie A. Fast, Stephen Fry, Carrie Fisher and Patty Duke.

Why?

The main reason I so respect these people is the work they have done to increase the positive public profile of bipolar disorder, but

---

[831] Forbes, 2015; Miller, 2009:179.

also just how much they managed to achieve in spite or because of their bipolar disorder. Obviously many people have heard of three of my idols as they have their own very public profiles, but you may not have heard of Kay Redfield Jamison and Julie Fast. Dr Kay Redfield Jamison and Julie Fast are my number top of the top bipolar idols.

Kay Redfield Jamison

Not only is Kay Redfield Jamison herself bipolar but she is also a leading researcher in bipolar studies. She is a Professor of Psychiatry at John Hopkins University. She has written and co-authored several books and treatises, my favourite being her stunningly written autobiographical work *An Unquiet Mind*. It is a beautiful story of her phenomenal journey with bipolar disorder; I recommend it as a great read to anyone, not just those with bipolar. She is amazing, formidable and inspiring. I would love one day to meet her and thank her for the positive impact she has had on my life.

Julie A. Fast

Julie Fast is herself BPII, and her husband of ten years is BPI. She is a prolific writer, blogger, contributor to bphope.com and a marvellous public speaker. She is truly inspirational in many ways. If I could be the next Julie Fast, I would consider my life to have been truly worth something. I have so much love for this woman who's book *Loving Someone with Bipolar Disorder* is one of my favourite bipolar books and was so helpful to me when I had a new diagnosis. She is phenomenal.

Stephen Fry

Stephen Fry has long been a household name around the globe. He is known for his wit, intelligence and sardonic humour. Now he is also known for the fact he has cyclothymia, a form of bipolar which is widely underestimated in its impact on a person's life. Stephen

Fry is a prolific actor, presenter and author, but he is also a supporter of those with mental health problems. I thoroughly enjoyed reading his autobiographies and adore watching him on programmes like QI and Blackadder. I am also so grateful to him for sharing his story with the world; he has given hope to people like me and knowledge to everyone who reads his works.

Carrie Fisher

Carrie Fisher is probably best known for her role in the Star Wars films, but she is also known for her continuous struggles with bipolar disorder and substance abuse. Her work with mental health charities and her hilariously witty autobiography helped raise the profile of bipolar disorder quite dramatically and I am sad that I will never be able to thank her.

Patty Duke

Patty Duke was a renowned actor. She is one of the first people in the public eye to have been open about what was at the time called manic-depressive illness. Her fabulous book with Gloria Hochman, *A Glorious Madness,* is the perfect marriage of textbook and autobiography and helped me to consider the format of my own book. I am in her debt.

So those are my Bipolar Idols.

Bipolar: friend or foe?

For me, a lot of the time my bipolar feels like the enemy; when I am depressed or overly sensitive or irritable I hate my bipolar. Often I wish I didn't have bipolar; I wouldn't have had to endure my crippling depressions, I wouldn't have felt suicidal, I wouldn't have had to pick up the pieces after sexual indiscretions or deal with the backlash of hypomanic spending sprees. Maybe if I didn't have bipolar disorder I could live a normal life with normal problems. Of course maybe I'd still have gotten depressed, still have been careless with money, still have cheated on partners. But I know my bipolar has played a part in all these things.

Sometimes I am glad I have bipolar disorder. It has taught me an empathy that cannot be learnt without having suffered yourself. Bipolar hypomania has helped me to achieve some great things. I have been made to feel overjoyed and full of life in a way that few in the world get to experience. Bipolar has shown me that I need to enjoy the small things, appreciate the little victories and trust in people. Without the pain that I have suffered I may not know the value of friends and family in the way that I do. Without my indiscretions I might not be able to forgive so readily. Without my mood swings I might not have been able to appreciate the importance of peace and quiet.

Sometimes I view bipolar as something completely separate from myself; as an external entity forcing its will on me. I see bipolar as a foe to be reckoned with, something to argue against; a metaphysical being to be fought away or conquered.

Sometimes I view bipolar as my whole being; a force inside of myself which has taken me over and is the driver in my vehicular body. Sometimes I think of myself as nothing but an incarnation of my bipolar with no separate identity; completely overrun by the strength of a power from which I cannot be extricated.

But bipolar is all and none of the above. You cannot simply conquer bipolar, you cannot simply celebrate it. Bipolar disorder is not outside of me, nor is it my entire definition. Bipolar is not a friend to love or a foe to fight. Bipolar is a facet of my many-faced identity. It is an obstacle and a light. Some say bipolar disorder is a gift, I think that ignores its destructive power. Some call it a curse, I think this ignores the boundless potential it grants us. I believe living with bipolar presents opportunities to learn. It gives us trials to overcome, but it also gives us euphoria to appreciate.

No, bipolar is not a friend. Bipolar is not a foe. Bipolar is a part of us we must live with, a housemate to negotiate and share with. Bipolar is a strong force within ourselves which teaches resilience like nothing else. It teaches us to love and care for others like nothing else. It teaches us to be strong. Bipolar teaches us to be flexible. I suppose I believe that bipolar is a teacher before it is anything else. And so, although I do still wish sometimes that I didn't have bipolar, I choose to be grateful for the lessons I have learnt as a result of having this disorder. I hope you too can feel this way.

A Marathon of Sprints and Stops

As already discussed getting and staying stable is hard work. It takes a lot of gusto to try every day to reach the goal of stability. I read once that as long as we persevere and try anything in the quest for balance and wellness, then we are heroes. In my opinion that's a touch of hyperbole, but I get the sentiment. It's hard work and as long as we keep pushing, keep striving for stability then we're doing well. My psychotherapist is always encouraging me to focus on the process and progress, so if you're still getting there, you're doing amazingly. Remember that.

I compare the road to stability with a marathon.

First, for most people running a marathon is about achieving a personal goal. Athletes may run to beat everyone else, but regular people run to complete the course, to win for themselves. When you have bipolar you are running to reach your own goal, running for yourself.

Second, it's a slog. No one finds a marathon easy, even walking it is hard work. So too is trying to get stable with bipolar; it is a slog, it takes a lot of determination, resilience and practice.

Third is training. No one can run a marathon without training; they jog up and down hills, they walk for miles, they take care of their feet and find the right training shoes for them. In bipolar we train ourselves to achieve sustained wellness. We find the right tools to help us, we practise the techniques we need to manage and survive, we can't just run the marathon without these things.

Fourth, it takes a long time. The marathon is not like other athletic events, it takes endurance to last the time it takes to run. With bipolar you need endurance to reach stability.

Fifth, as a regular person, it is difficult to just run the whole way, it's impossible to sprint from start to finish. You may start off with a quick sprint from the starting line; so too with bipolar on your journey to wellness you may make a great bound at the start. Then you need to slow your pace; with bipolar you jog a lot, rather than run. And from time to time, you walk. It means sometimes you have to slow down your progress so the target is achievable. You can't go hell-for-leather the whole time else you'll flag too often and burn yourself out too many times.

Sixth, sometimes when you're running a marathon you have to stop to catch your breath. When you're striving for stability you have to sometimes stop and take a breather, acknowledge you need to stop for a little while; so pause and appreciate the progress you've made so far. No matter how far you've run, you've done great to get this far.

Finally, you have to replenish your energy. Even the athletes take on water and eat energy bars whilst they're running. From time to time you need to do things that recharge you; enjoy the fruits of your labours and get the energy to allow you to carry on. You can't keep running if you're dehydrated.

So you see, getting stable is like a marathon filled with all its requisite steps.

A Reason, Not an Excuse
This is something I feel very strongly about.

Bipolar affects our behaviours

Because we have bipolar disorder our moods are often more extreme than others'. Because we have bipolar disorder our behaviours are often more erratic than others'. Sometimes our moods and behaviours cause discomfort or harm to others. There are two ways we can respond when how we have been has had a negative impact on others; one is okay, the other definitely isn't. One is, 'I'm sorry that I hurt you, I was having an episode and was not in full control. I will endeavour to do more to protect you from my episodes in the future'. The other is, 'It's not my fault, I have bipolar disorder'. Can you guess which is okay? Now obviously that's a bit black and white, I'm sure there are shades between the two, but the main point remains. In one you apologise for your behaviour, in the other you don't; in one you accept the blame, in the other you don't.

The point I'm trying to make is given in the title of this section. Having bipolar may be a reason for the way we are sometimes, but it is not an excuse. We must still accept responsibility for our actions, even if we were not in our right mind. It is not acceptable to simply blame bipolar every time we do something wrong. It is not okay to think all will be forgiven if we wave the bipolar flag. It is not allowable to deliberately undertake actions which are dangerous or unkind and then later write it off to bipolar. Remember, 'bipolar is a part of me, it is not my defining feature'. Everyone does stupid things from time to time, they just apologise, accepting that what they did was wrong. We must do the same.

Now you can apologise and still recognise that your bipolar had something to do with your behaviour. You can say, I have said, 'I'm sorry I hurt your feelings, I did not do it deliberately. I was depressed and did not think of how my actions would affect you'. You are letting that person know that, in your opinion, bipolar played a part, but you are still apologising and taking ownership of what happened.

It's worth noting that apologising does not automatically mean you are forgiven, straightaway or even at all. If that is the case, it is still not alright to play the bipolar card. It is unlikely to make people forgive you if you foist the blame elsewhere. It's like telling your mum your brother made you do it. It doesn't stop her being angry with you, now she's just angry at him too. So too, if you blame your mental health with a 'bipolar made me do it', the person you've hurt is likely to just get more upset. Best simply to apologise again and give them some space (tell them you're giving them space!).

Sharing the blame

Bipolar is only a part of us. Bipolar is not our defining feature: If we start to blame bipolar for all our misbehaviours then we have to start crediting our bipolar with all of our achievements as well. We work hard for our successes, why would we want to cede ownership to our bipolar? It doesn't make any sense; we wouldn't. No one would think we were being fair to ourselves if we said, 'Well I can't take any credit, I've been hypomanic all week'. Well if we're not going to blame our bipolar when we do well, we can't blame our bipolar when we do poorly. We owe it to people to be sincere and honest; we owe it to ourselves.

Stability is the Goal
The Goal:

As we know, BPII is not curable, but it is manageable. At the crux of the matter is stability. What most of us with BPII want more than anything is stability. 'The overall goal is for [us] to get healthy and stay healthy'.[832] Stability is the goal.[833]

Why? Because bipolar symptoms and mood episodes generally have a negative impact on our lives. Whereas a reduction of bipolar symptoms and an overall stable mood promotes 'Positive health benefits ... Greater satisfaction and enjoyment ... Clear thinking ... Good behaviour ... Better relationships ... Strong libido ... Solid resilience ... The ability to overcome personal barriers ... A great sense of wellbeing ... Physical health benefits ... Better management of your physical health ... [and] Economic benefits'.[834] Stability is our best possible state.

Stability does not necessarily mean the complete elimination of symptoms and mood states, but it does mean better coping and a greater resilience against episodes and symptoms.

Lifestyle:

We have already discussed many lifestyle choices which can have a dramatically positive effect on our mental state and on our ability to control or overcome our symptoms. There is a lot we can do to help ourselves, it's 'not just about medication'.[835]

'Structuring your life is a very important aspect of mood hygiene'.[836] Mood hygiene being those things we do to keep bipolar episodes at bay. A strong daily routine can help keep symptoms from occurring.[837] This may include regular sleep schedules,[838] keeping your mind focused (not just relaxing it),[839] regular meal times,[840]

---

[832] White, 2014:8.
[833] Jackel, 2010.
[834] Miller, 2009:27-29.
[835] Paquette, 2016.
[836] Mondimore, 1999:226.
[837] NCCMH, 2006:395.
[838] Roberts et al., 2013:50; Miller, 2009:107; Fieve, 2006:108; NCCMH, 2006:375.
[839] Miller, 2009:107.
[840] Roberts et al., 2013:50.

finding the right job or choosing not to work,[841] and maintaining optimal levels of activity and exercise.[842]

Many people with bipolar disorder emphasise the role of routine and schedule in maintaining stability.[843] Identifying and avoiding triggers and a few simple lifestyle changes, such as limiting your alcohol intake,[844] can have a dramatic impact on staying well.[845] Though it is worth noting that it is unlikely that lifestyle changes and improved stress management will stop all bipolar symptoms from arising completely.[846]

Here is my list of positive lifestyle choices and good coping skills for staying stable with BPII:

- Take your meds as prescribed.[847]
- Exercise as much as you are able.[848]
- Record your moods.[849]
- Get plenty of sunlight, especially in the winter.[850]
- Learn skills to manage stress and conflict.[851]
- Get plenty of relaxation time.
- Keep your brain active.[852]
- Use your support network.[853]
- Work through self-help books.
- Keep your appointments with doctors, psychotherapists, etc.[854]

---

[841] Haycock, 2010:131-136.
[842] Roberts et al., 2013:50.
[843] Roberts et al., 2013:50; Kennard, 2011:23; Mondimore, 1999:222 & 226.
[844] Mondimore, 1999:227.
[845] NCCMH, 2006:375.
[846] NCCMH, 2006:296.
[847] NCCMH, 2006:102; Mondimore, 1999:225.
[848] NHS, 2016; Lamden, 2014.
[849] Mondimore, 1999:227.
[850] Miller, 2009:32.
[851] Lamden, 2014; NCCMH, 2006:102; Mondimore, 1999:226.
[852] Miller, 2009:107.
[853] NCCMH, 2006:102.

- Accept your diagnosis.[855]
- Come to terms with what you may have lost due to your bipolar and create new targets and dreams.[856]
- Meditate or practise mindfulness.
- Create a self-management programme using advice from your mental health team and self-help books.[857]
- Cut negative people from your life.[858]
- Maintain a healthy diet.
- Avoid drugs.[859]
- Identify mood triggers.[860]
- Focus on things that are meaningful to you.[861]
- Socialise.
- Get plenty of sleep.[862]
- Make big changes if necessary, like quitting your job, declaring bankruptcy or delaying a wedding.[863]
- Get educated about BPII.[864]
- Don't procrastinate at all, not over important nor over trivial things.[865]

Remember '[r]elapse prevention is suicide prevention' too.[866] So every little thing you do that keeps you away from depression and mixed episodes, subsequently helps keep you away from suicide.

Prodromes:

One of the most integral coping mechanisms to help nip in the bud

---

[854] Fieve, 2006:232.
[855] NCCMH, 2006:102.
[856] Fast & Preston, 2012:197.
[857] NHS, 2016.
[858] Haycock, 2010:136-138.
[859] Lamden, 2014.
[860] McManamy, 2006:172; NCCMH, 2006:102.
[861] Boyes, 2015:47.
[862] NCCMH, 2006:102.
[863] Mondimore, 1999:226,
[864] NCCMH, 2006:102.
[865] Mondimore, 1999:227.
[866] Mondimore, 1999:238.

any mood episodes is recognition of and action upon the onset of early warning signs and symptoms, known as prodromes. Poor coping strategies in response to prodromes has been linked with an increase in relapse.[867] It is crucial to stability that you catch a bipolar episode from the very first symptoms if you're going to head it off successfully.[868] Of course at the beginning of your bipolar you won't necessarily know what symptoms to look out for as early warning signs of an impending episode (though you could consider the lists of symptoms from earlier in the book). However, over time we all develop some knowledge of our prodromes and we are often able to identify them.[869] It is important that we learn our own prodromes as they are a pattern unique to us and our illness.[870] Learning to spot our prodromes gives us some control over the course of our disorder, because early recognition leads to early intervention.

That being said, it can be difficult to recognise prodromes, especially of depression. One study revealed that 25% of those with bipolar struggled to identify warning signs of depression versus just 7.5% saying they could not recognise prodromes of mania and hypomania.[871] I reckon this is because some common prodromes of depression are less noticeable or easier to write off; like feeling tired, eating more and getting easily stressed. It's easier to notice when you are feeling electric, not eating and performing especially well at work. So, it's more obvious to us when we are entering a hypomanic state.[872] Also, in my experience, hypomanias come on much more quickly than depressions.

Triggers:

Aside from prodromes, recognising triggers and learning how to

---

[867] Kennard, 2011:26.
[868] Fast & Preston, 2012:66.
[869] Kennard, 2011:20; Fieve, 2006:232; Lam & Wong, 1997.
[870] NCCMH, 2006:98 & 357.
[871] Lam & Wong, 1997.
[872] NCCMH, 2006:357.

mitigate or avoid them is a key aspect of staying well. It is important to remember that while not all relapses have obvious triggers,[873] noticing triggers where they are evident has a dramatic effect on our ability to stay well. In particular, stress is a common trigger (as discussed earlier)[874] and anything we do to reduce or eliminate stress can only have positive effects on our mental well-being and our ability to prevent or reduce the number of mood episodes we experience.

Learning our triggers is a lifelong process, but if we pay attention to and reflect upon which environmental triggers brought on episodes early in our illness, when they are more prevalent,[875] then it becomes an easier task. Recognising triggers from early in the development of our disorder is key to avoiding similar triggers as time goes on.

Of course, some potential triggers simply cannot be avoided, such as the death or marriage of a loved one. And despite the preventative measures we put in place, daily stresses are still likely to occur; stress can just happen, and life must still go on. Other contributing factors like inter-episode depressive symptoms, comorbid anxiety or drug misuse can be approached and their effects reduced through psychotherapies, improving '[q]uality of life, function and disability'.[876]

The Aim:

And I think I'll end this section on a quote from the NCCMH:

> 'The effects of lifestyle in people with bipolar disorder are not confined to considerations about the onset of bipolar disorder, the onset and recovery from manic and

---

[873] NCCMH, 2006:99.
[874] Mondimore, 1999:224.
[875] Mondimore, 1999:224.
[876] NCCMH, 2006:377.

depressive episodes, and the prevention of suicide. While these outcomes tend to be, and probably should remain, the most important issues in the mind of many healthcare professionals, there are other important considerations in the minds of people with bipolar disorder and their carers. Issues that are important to people with bipolar disorder include social adjustment and function, quality of life, physical health and appearance, spiritual life, the life of carers and family, issues of personal control over their life, stigma and finances.'[877]

If you're reading this book because it's a loved one who has BPII

Thank you. It makes such a huge difference when the people who love us choose to educate themselves. So, a massive thank you. Reading this book has hopefully given you some insight into what life feels like for us. Hopefully it hasn't scared you too much or given you even more reasons for concern. But it is important for you to know what it's like for us, and everything I've included in this book is good to know whether it is you or a loved one with BPII. It really can make the world of difference to be educated about the condition by more than the DSM-IV.

Some advice

- Well you're already doing number one: learn. Learn about bipolar disorder from books, from websites and from blogs. Learn as much as you can. Understanding a little of what your loved one goes through, how they might feel and think helps them and it helps you. Keep learning; I have a tonne of recommendations at the end of the book.
- Talk about bipolar. Especially talk to your loved one. They need to know their disorder is not a taboo topic; that

[877] NCCMH, 2006:376.

you're not scared of talking about it. Ask them to explain how they're feeling when they can. Ask them what they think when they're in a mood episode. Ask them how they feel about their bipolar. Learn from them about <u>their</u> bipolar disorder.

- Pay attention to the signals. Sometimes we don't realise we're entering into a mood state, if you see the signs tell us. Ask us to go to the doctor or call the clinic. You can help us manage our bipolar just by pointing out when we should get help from our mental health team.
- Look out for warning signs that things are really bad. You need to agree this with your loved one when they are stable(ish), but you may need to intervene on their behalf. If you've discussed this when they are of sound mind, you may want to call the mental health team if you're worried. You may even have in place an arrangement, in an Advanced Directive, where you can ask for your loved one to be admitted to hospital in extreme moods states. You need to tell your loved one if you see dangerous signs that they are unwell, but you may also need to tell their CPN, GP, social worker, or psychiatry team. It is in their best interest and paramount to their safety.
- Take care of yourself! You cannot always be there 100%, you cannot give all your time and energy to looking after your loved one. You have to take time out for yourself. It is good to have a space that is physically your own where you can go to recharge and relax. Remember to still do things for yourself; all the tips from the 'Stability is the Goal' and 'Wasting Time with a Purpose' sections apply to you too. You have to stay well and energised; taking care of or looking out for someone with bipolar disorder can be draining both physically and emotionally.
- Most importantly, build your own support network. Your loved one may need you to talk to and to help them, but

you also need people to talk to and to help you. Find people you can talk to when you're tired, concerned or need help. You can talk to your loved one's CPN or social worker, but you should have people who are just your own. Friends and family who aren't also involved in the support network of your bipolar loved one may be best. You could also consider a counsellor or therapist so you can talk to a professional to help you work through issues or tackle problems. You could do just a few sessions if things are tough, or you could have regular appointments; you <u>are</u> allowed.

Thank you

Thank you on behalf of your loved one for learning about BPII. But also thank you from me; the more people who are educated about bipolar disorder the less scary and more accepted it becomes. So thank you from the bottom of my heart, you are genuinely helping to change the world and their view of bipolar disorder.

Thank you

Thank You and Goodbye

And with that we come to the end of the book.

Let me start by saying thank you. Thank you for reading 'Life with Bipolar Type Two'. This book was written for you and without you it is meaningless and purposeless. My aim was to educate and support those with BPII; I hope that I have achieved this. I hope that in reading my book you have learnt something you didn't know and gleaned some ideas on how to live stably with BPII.

In researching and writing this book I have not only learnt a lot about BPII in general, but I have also learnt a lot about my bipolar. It has caused me to reflect on my experiences and symptoms and led to my garnering new insight into my bipolar disorder. I hope that 'Life with Bipolar Type Two' has given you pause at times and caused you too to reflect on your own bipolar.

Further, I hope that I have offered you some sound guidance with which to create a wellness management plan and make informed lifestyle choices. Don't forget, a few small changes are often not only more achievable, but also more beneficial in the long run than a grand redesigning of our whole lives. I don't always do everything I have suggested in these pages, but what I do I am consistent with. And I am slowly introducing more and more of the techniques I have presented. I am not a paragon of stability, but I am still working on it. Every day.

And, finally, thank you again. I have put a lot into this book, and it was all for you. I hope it has helped.

Goodbye, and good luck on your bipolar journey.

Eleanor x

Bibliography

Recommended reading

Duke, P. & Hochman, G. 1992. *A Brilliant Madness, Living with Manic-Depressive Illness.* Bantam Books: New York, NY.

Fast, J. A. & Preston, J. D. 2012. *loving someone with bipolar disorder.* New Harbinger Publications: Oakland, CA.

Fieve, R. R. 2006. *Bipolar II.* Rodale:New York, NY.

Fink, C & J. 2005. *Bipolar Disorder for Dummies.* John Wiley Publishing: New York NY.

Fisher, C. 2008. *Wishful Drinking.* Pocket Books: London.

Flanigan, R. 2016. *Bipolar & Mindfulness: Bringing Back Balance.* http://www.bphope.com [accessed 05.08.17].

Fletcher, J. 2017. *Bipolar Disorder: Signs, symptoms, and diagnosis.* Medical News Today. http://www.medicalnewstoday.com/articles/318124.php [accessed 05.08.17].

Fry, S. 2010. *The Fry Chronicles.* Penguin: London.

Fry, S. 2014. *More Fool Me.* Penguin: London.

Haycock, D. A. 2010. *The Everything Health Guide to Adult Bipolar Disorder.* Adams Media: Anon, MA.

Hodges, L. 2012. *Living with Bipolar Disorder: Strategies for Balance and Resilience.* Findhorn Press: Forres.

Mondimore, F. M. 2006. *Bipolar Disorder: A Guide for Patients and Families.* John Hopkins University Press.

Owen, S. & Saunders, A. 2008. *Bipolar Disorder: The Ultimate Guide.* One World Publications.

Redfield Jamison, K. 1993. *Touched with Fire: Manic Depressive Illness and the Artistic Temperament.* Free Press: New York, NY.

Redfield Jamison, K. 1995. *An Unquiet Mind.* Alfred A Knopf: New York, NY.

Redfield Jamison, K. 2000. *Night Falls Fast.* Vintage Books: New York, NY.

Roberts, S. M et al. 2013. *The Bipolar II Disorder Workbook.* New Harbinger Publications: Oakland, CA.

Sandiou, A. 2017. *Bipolar Breakthrough: New Study Reveals Disease-Causing Mechanism.* Medical News Today. http://www.medicalnewstoday.com/articles/315914.php [accessed 05.08.17].

Resources I used for research

Albrecht, A. T. & Herrick, C. 2007. *100 Questions and Answers About Bipolar Disorder.* Jones and Bartlett Publishers: Burlington, MA.

Baek, J. H., Park, D. Y., Choi, J., Kim, J. S., Choi, J. S., Ha, K., Kwon, J. S., Lee, D. & Hong, K. S. 2011. 'Differences Between Bipolar I and Bipolar II Disorders in Clinical Features, Comorbidity, and Family History.' (abstract) *Journal of Affective Disorders,* 131(1-3): 59-67.

Baglioni, C., Battaliese, G., Feige, B. S., Spiegelhalder, K., Nissen, C., Voderholzer, U., Lombardo, C. & Riemann, D. 2011. 'Insomnia as a Preictor of Depression: A Meta-analytical Evaluation of Longitudinal Epidemiological Studies.' (abstract) *Journal of Affective Disorders,* 135:10-19.

Ball, A. R., Mitchell, P.B., Corry, J. C., Skillecorn, A., Smith, M. & Mahli, G. S. 2006. 'A Randomized Controlled Trial of Cognitive Therapy for Bipolar Disorder: Focus on Long-Term Change.' (abstract) *Journal of Clinical Psychiatry* 67(2): 277-286.

Barlow, D. H., Allen, L. B. & Choate, M. L. 2004. 'Towards a Unified Treatment for Emotional Disorders.' (abstract) *Behaviour Therapy,* 35(2):205-230.

Bauer, M. S., Callahan, A. M., Jampala, C., Petty, F., Sajatoic, M., Schaefer, V., Wittlin, B. & Powell, B. J. 1999. 'Clinical Practice Guidelines for Bipolar Disorder from the Department of Veterans Affairs.' (abstract) *Journal of Clinical Psychiatry,* 60:9-21.

Bauer, M. S., McBride, L., Williford, W. O., Glick, H., Kinosian, B., Altshuler, L., Beresford, T., Kilbourne, A. M., Sajatovic, M.; Cooperative Studies Program 430. 2006. 'Collaborative care for bipolar disorder part II: impact on clinical outcome, function, and costs.' *Psychiatric Services,* 57(7):937-945.

Beckmann, H. 1983. 'Phenylalanine in Affective Disorders.' (abstract) *Advances in Biological Psychiatry,* 10:137-147.

Bipolar Lives. ... *Bipolar 2 is more common than you may realize.* http://www.bipolar-lives.com/bipolar-type-2.html. [accessed 12.08.17].

BipolarLab.com. *1.3.1.1 Criteria for a Manic/Hypomanic Episodes.* http://www.bipolarlab.com/index.php?option=com_content&view=article&id=48:maniccriteria&catid=21:bipolar&Itemid=77 [accessed 21.08.17]

Boerlin, H. L., Gitlin, M. J., Zoellner, L. A. & Hammen, C. L. 1998. 'Bipolar depression and antidepressant-induced mania: a naturalistic study.' (abstract) *Journal of Clinical Psychiatry,* 59:374-379.

Boyes, A. 2015. *The Anxiety Toolkit.* Piatkus: London.

bp Magazine. 2016. *The Bipolar Symptom Nobody Wants to Talk About.* http://www.bphope.com [accessed 05.08.17].

bp Magazine. 2017. *Talking to Yourself in the Third Person Can Help You Control Emotions.* http://www.bphope.com [accessed 05.08.17].

Brown, R. & Gerbarg, P. 2005. 'Sudarshan Kriya Yogic Breathing in the Treatment of Stress, Anxiety, and Depression: Part II – Clinical Applications and Guidelines.' *Journal of Alternative and Complementary Medicine,* 11 no4:711-717.

Byrne, A. & Byrne, D. G. 1993. 'The Effect of Exercise on Depression, Anxiety and other mood states: a review.' (abstract) *Journal of Psychosomatic Research,* 37:565-574.

Chang, K. D., Blasey, C., Ketter, T. A. & Steiner, H. 2001. 'Family Environment of Children and Adolescents with Bipolar Parents.' (abstract) *Bipolar Disorders,* 2:68-72.

Chellingsworth, M & Farrand, P. 2015. *How to Beat Depression One Step at a Time.* Robinson: London.

Chouinard, G., Youn, S. N. & Annable, L. 1985. 'A Controlled Clinical Trial of L-Tryptophan in Acute Mania.' (abstract) *Biological Psychiatry,* 20:546-547.

Chouinard, G., Young, S. N., Bradwejn, J. & Annable, L. 1983. 'Tryptophan in the treatment of depression and mania'. (abstract) *Advances in Biological Psychiatry,* 10:47-66.

Cochran, S. D. 1984. 'Preventing Medical Noncompliance in

Outpatient Treatment of Bipolar Affective Disorders.' (abstract) *Journal of Consulting and Clinical Psychology,* 52(5): 873-878.

Colom, F., Vieta, E., Martinez-Aran, A., Reinares, M., Goikolea, J. M., Benabarre, A., Torrent, C., Comes, M., Corbella, B., Parramon, G. & Corominas, J. 2003. 'A Randomized Trial on the Efficacy of Group Psychoeducation in the Prophylaxis of Recurrences in Bipolar Patients Whose Disease Is in Remission.' *Archives of General Psychiatry,* 60(4): 402-407.

Coryell, W., Solomon, D., Turvey, C., Keller, M., Leon, A. C., Endicott, J., Schettler, P., Judd, L. & Mueller, T. 2003. 'The long-term course of rapid-cycling bipolar disorder.' *Archives of General Psychiatry,* 60(9):914-920.

Craft, L. L. & Landers, D. M. 1998. 'The effects of exercise on clinical depression and depression resulting from mental illness: a meta-regression analysis.' (abstract) *Journal of Sports and Exercise Psychology,* 20:339-357.

Dawson, M. 2006. *Bipolar & Sleep: Problems and Solutions.* http://www.bphope.com [accessed 05.08.17].

Deckersbach, T., Hölzel, B. K., Eisner, L. R., Stange, J. P., Peckham, A. D., Dougherty, D. D., Rauch, S. L., Lazar, S. & Nierenberg, A. A. 2012. 'Mindfulness-Based Cognitive Therapy for Nonremitted Patients with Bipolar Disorder.' (abstract) *CNS Neuroscience and Therapeutics,* 18(2): 133-141.

Deckersbach, T., Perlis, R. H., Frankle, W. G., Gray, S. M., Grandin, L., Dougherty, D. D., Nierenberg, A. A. & Sachs, G. S. 2004. 'Presence of Iritability During Depressive Episodes in Bipolar Disorder.' (abstract) *CNS Spectrums,* 9(3):227-231.

Duke, P. & Hochman, G. 1993. *A Brilliant Madness, Living with Manic-Depressive Illness.* Bantam Books: New York, NY.

Dunner, D. 2003. 'Clinical Consequences of Under-Recognized Bipolar Spectrum Diorser.' (abstract) *Bipolar Disorders,* 5:456-463.

Eriksson, S. & Gard, G. 2011. 'Physical Exercise and Depression'. *Physical Therapy Reviews,* 16:261-268.

Fast, J. A. 2006. *Straight Talk About Suicide.* http://www.bphope.com [accessed 05.08.17].

Fast, J. 2014. *Double Trouble: Physical Pain & Bipolar's "Psychic Pain".* http://bphope.com [accessed 07.08.17].

Fisher, C. 2008. *Wishful Drinking.* Simon & Schuster: London.

Flanigan, R. I. 2016. 'Biplar & Mindfulness: Bringing Back Balance'. *bpHope Magazine.*

Fogarty, E. 2013. *Diary of a Bipolar Survivor.* Chipmunkapublishing: Brentwood.

Forbes, E. 2015. *Pets & Bipolar: Friends with Benefits.* http://www.bphope.com [accessed 05.08.17].

Frank, E., Gonzalez, J. M. & Fagiolini, A. 2006. 'The Importance of Routine for Preventing Recurrence in Bipolar Disorder.' *American Journal of Psychiatry,* 163:981-985.

Freeman, M. P., Hibbeln, J. R., Wisner, K. L., Davis, J. M., Mischoulon, D., Peet, M., Keck, P. E., Marangell, L. B., Richardson, A. J. Lake, J. & Stoll, A. L. 2006. 'Omega-3 Fatty Acids: Evidence Basis for Treatment and Future Research in Psychiatry'. *Journal of Clinical Psychiatry,* 67:1954-1967.

Ghaemi, S. N. 2008. 'Treatment of rapid-cycling bipolar disorder: Are antidepressants mood destabilizers?' *The American Journal of Psychiatry,* 165(3): 300-302.

Ghaemi, S. N., Lenox, M. S. & Baldessarini, R. J. 2001 'Effectiveness and safety of long0term antidepressant treatment in bipolar disorder.' (abstract) *Journal of Clinical Psychiatry,* 62:565-569.

Glenister, D. 1996. 'Exercise and Mental Health: a review.' (abstract) *Journal of the Royal Society of Health,* 116:7-13.

Goldstein, T. R., Axelson, D. A. Birmaher, B. & Brent, D. A. 2007. 'Dialectal Behaviour Therapy for Adolescents with Bipolar Disorder: A 1-Year Open Trial.' (abstract) *Journal of the American Academy of Child & Adolescent Psychiatry,* 46(7):820-830.

Grandin, L. D., Alloy, L. B. & Abramson, L.Y. 2006. 'The Social Zeitberger Theory, Circadian Rhythms, and Mood Disorders: Review and Evaluation.' (abstract) *Clinical Psychology Review,* 26(6): 679-694.

Gray, S. M. & Otto, M. W. 2001. 'Psychosocial approaches to suicide prevention: applications to patients with bipolar disorder.' (abstract) *Journal of Clinical Psychiatry,* 62(25):56-64.

Gruber, J. M., Miklowitz, D. J., Harvey, A. G., Frank, E., Kupfer, D., Thase, M. E., Sachs, G.s . & Ketter, T. A. 2011.'Sleep Matters: Sleep, Functioning and Course of Illness in Bipolar Disorder.' (abstract) *Journal of Affective Disorders,* 134:416-420.

Hall-Flavin. D. K. 2012. *Bipolar medications and weaight gain.* http://www.mayoclinic.com/health/bipolar-medications-and-weight-gain/AN02062 [accessed 04.05.2018]

Harkavy-Friedman, J. M, Keilp, J. G., Grunebaum, M. F., Sher, L., Printz, D., Burke, A. K., Mann, J. J. & Oquendo, M. 2006. 'Are BPI and BPII suicide attempters distinct neuropsychologically?' *Journal of Affective Disorders,* 94 (1-3):255-259.

Health Line. *Diagnosis Guide for Bipolar Disorder.* http://www.healthline.com/health/bipolar-disorder/bipolar-diagnosis-guide#Mentalhealthevaluation3 [accessed 21.08.17]

Himmelhoch, J. M. 1998. 'Social anxiety, hypomania and the bipolar spectrum: data, theory and clinical issues.' (abstract) *Journal of Affective Disorders,* 50:203-213.

Hlastala, S. A., Frank, E., Mallinger, A. G., Thase, M. E., Ritenour, A. M. & Kupfer, D. J. 1997. 'Bipolar Depression: an underestimated treatment challenge.' (abstract) *Depression and Anxiety,* 5:73-83.

Hong, J., Reed, C., Novick, D., Haro, J. M. & Aguado, J. 2011. 'Clinical and Economic Consequences of Medication Non-adherence in the Treatment of Patients with Manic/Mixed Episode of Bipolar Disorder: Results from the European Mania in Bipolar Longitudinal Evaluation of Medication (EMBLEM) study.' (abstract) *Psychiatry Research,* 190:110-114.

Hornbacher, M. 2008. *Madness, A Bipolar Life.* Houghton Mifflin: Boston, MA.

Jackel, Donna. 2010. *Everything You Ever Wanted To Know About BIPOLAR DEPRESSION.* http://www.bphope.com [accessed 25.08.17].

Jamison, K. R. 1995. 'Manic-Depressive Illness and Creativity.' *Scientific American,* 64 (Feb 1995).

Johnson, J. 2016. *Bipolar Disorder and Alcohol: What's the Connection?* Medical News Today. http://www.medicalnewstoday.com/articles/313571.php [accessed 05.08.17].

Johnson, S. L. 2005. 'Life Events in Bipolar Disorder: Towards

More Specific Models.' (abstract) *Clinical Psychology Review,* 117(2): 268-277.

Johnson, S. 2017. *Are Pets A Secret Weapon When Battling Bipolar Disorder?* http://www.bphope.com [accessed 05.08.17].

Jónsdóttir, H., Opjordsmoen, S., Birkenaes, A. B., Simonsen, C., Engh, J. A., Ringen, P. A., Vaskinn, A., Friis, S., Sundet, K. & Andreassen, O. A. 2013. 'Predictors of Medication Adherence in Patients with Schizophrenia and Bipolar Disorder.' (abstract) *Acta Psychiatrica Scandivica,* 127:23-33.

Judd, L. L., Akiskal, H. S., Schettler, P. J., Endicott, J., Maser, J., Solomon, D. A., Leon, A. C. & Keller, M. B. 2003. 'A prospective investigation of the natural history of the long-term weekly symptomatic status of bipolar II disorder.' (abstract) *Archives of General Psychiatry,* 60:261-269.

Kennard, J. 2011. *Bipolar Disorder: a short introductory guide.* Amazon.

Kessler, R. C., Chiu, W. T., Demler, O. & Walters, E. E. 2005. 'Prevalence, Severity, and Comorbidity of 12-month DSM-IV Disorders in the National Comorbidity Survey Replication.' *Archives of General Psychiatry,* 62(6):617-627.

Khamba, B., Aucoin, M., Tsirgielis, D., Copeland, A., Vermani, M., Cameron, C., Szpindel, I., Laidlaw, B., Epstein, I. & Katzman, M. 2011. 'Effectiveness of Vitamin D in the Treatment of Mood Disorders: A Literature Review.' *Journal of Orthomolecular Medicine,* 26:127-135.

Kilbourne, A. M., Rofey, D. L., McCarthy, J. F., Post, E. P., Welsh, D. & Blow, F. C. 2007. 'Nutrition and Exercise Behavior Among Patients with Bipolar Disorder.' (abstract) *Bipolar Disorders,*

9(5):443-452.

Krueger, A. 2017. *Why Bipolar Disorder is So Hard to Diagnose, and What You Can Do About It.* http://www.bphope.com [accessed 05.08.17]

Krueger, R. F. 1999. 'The structure of common mental disorders.' *Archives of General Psychiatry,* 56:921-926.

La Fontaine, T. P., Di Lorenzo, T. M., Frensch, P. A., Stucky-Ropp, R.C., Bargman, E. P. & McDonald, D. G. 1992. 'Aerobic exercise and mood.' (conclusion) *Sports medicine,* 13:160-170.

Lam, D.H., Hayward, P., Watkins, E.R., Wright, K. & Sham, P. 2005. 'Relapse Prevention in Patients with Bipolar Disorder: Cognitive Therapy Outcome After 2 Years.' *American Journal of Psychiatry,* 162(2): 324-329.

Lam, D. & Wong, G. 1997. 'Prodromes, coping strategies, insight and social functioning in bipolar affective disorders.' (abstract) *Psychological Medicine,* 27:1091-1100.

Lawlor, D. A. & Hopker, S. W. 2001. 'The Effectiveness of Exercise as an Intervention in the Management of Depression: Systematic Review and Meta-Regression Analysis of Randomised Controlled Trials.' *British Medical Journal,* 322(7289): 763-767.

Leader, D. 2013. *Strictly Bipolar.* Penguin: London.

Lepore, S. J. 1997. 'Expressive writing moderates the relation between intrusive thoughts and depressive symptoms.' *Journal of Personality and Social Psychology,* 73:1030-1037.

Linehan, M. M., Comtois, K. A., Murray, A. M., Brown, M. Z., Gallop, R. J., Heard, H. L., Korslund, K. E., Titek, D. A. Reynolds. S. K. & Lindenboim, N. 2006. 'Two-Year Randomized Controlled

Trial and Follow-up of Dialectal Behavior Therapy vs Therapy by Experts for Suicidal Behaviors and Borderline Personality Disorder.' *Archives of General Psychiatry,* 63(7): 757-766.

Liperoti, R., Landi, F., Fusco, O., Bernabei, R. & Onder, G. 2009. 'Omega-3 Polyunsaturated Fatty Acids and Depression: A Review of the Evidence.' (abstract) *Current Pharmaceutical Design,* 15:4165-4172.

Ma, S.H. & Teasdale, J. D. 2004.'Mindfulness-Based Cognitive Therapy for Depression: Replication and Exploration of Differential Relapse Prevention Effects.' (abstract) *Journal of Consulting and Clinical Psychology,* 72(1): 31-40.

MacGill, M. 2016. *How does Bipolar Disorder Affect Memory?* Medical News Today.
http://www.medicalnewstoday.com/articles/314328.php [accessed 05.08.17].

Marohn, S. 2008. *The Natural Medicine Guide to Bipolar Disorder.* Hampton Roads Publishing: Charlottesville, VA.

Mehta, F. 2016. *Bipolar Disorder: What is Rapid Cycling?* Medical News Today.
http://www.medicalnewstoday.com/articles/314093.php [accessed 05.08.17].

Miklowitz, D. J., Axelson, D. A., Birmaher, B., George, E. L., Taylor, D. O., Schneck, C. D., Beresford, C. A., Dickinson, L. M., Craighead, W. E.& Brent, D. A. 2008. 'Family-Focused Treatment for Adolescents with Bipolar Disorder: Results of a 2-Year Randomized Trial.' *Archives of General Psychiatry,* 65(9): 1053-1061.

Miklowitz, D. J., Otto, M. W., Frank, E., Reilly-Harrington, N. A., Kogan, J. N., Sachs, G. S., *et al.* 2007(a). 'Intensive Psychosocial

Intervention Enhances Functioning in Patients with Bipolar Depression: Results from a 9-Month Randomized Controlled Trial.' *American Journal of Psychiatry,* 164(9): 1340-1347.

Miklowitz, D. J., Otto, M. W., Frank, E., Reilly-Harrington, N. A., Wisniewski, S. R., Kogan, J. N. *et al.* 2007(b) 'Psychosocial Treatments for Bipolar Depression: A 1-Year Randomized Trial from the Systematic Treatment Enhancement Program.' *Archives of General Psychiatry,* 64(4):419-426.

Miklowitz, D. J., Simoneau, T. L., George, E. L., Richards, J. A., Kalbag, A., Sachs-Ericsson, N. & Suddath, R. 2000. 'Family-Focused Treatment of Bipolar Disorder: 1-Year Effects of a Psychoeducational Program in Conjunction with Pharmacotherapy.' (abstract) *Biological Psychiatry,* 48(6): 582-592.

Miller, L. 2009. *MoodMapping.* Rodale: London.

Moezzi, M. 2016. 'Bipolar Depression & Suicide – Gone Too Soon'. *bpHope Magazine.*

Myers, J. E. & Thase, M. E. 2000. 'Anxiety in the patient with bipolar disorder: recognition, significance, and approaches to treatment.' (abstract) *Psychiatric Annals,* 30:456-464.

NCCMH (National Collaborating Centre for Mental Health). 2006. *Bipolar Disorder.* The British Psychological Society & The Royal College of Psychiatrists: Leicester & London.

Newman, T. 2017. *Bipolar disorder speeds up biological aging.* Medical News Today.
http://www.medicalnewstoday.com/articles/318658.php
[accessed 05.08.17].

NHS. 2016. Bipolar Disorder webpage.

https://www.nhs.uk/cnditions/bipolar-disorder [accessed 20.04.18]

NHS. 2018. '10 Tips to Beat Insomnia.' http://www.nhs.uk/Livewell/insomnia/Pages/insomniatips.aspx

Nichols, H. 2016. *Bipolar Disorder in Women: What You Need To Know.* Medical News Today. http://www.medicalnewstoday.com/articles/314924.php [accessed 05.08.17].

NIMH. 2018. Bipolar Disorder webpage. https://www.nimh.nih.gov/health/topics/bipolar-disorder/index.shtml [accessed 20.04.18]

Nolen-Hoeksema, S. & Morrow, J. 1991. 'A Prospective Study of Depression and Posttraumatic Stress Symptoms After a Natural Disaster: The 1989 Loma Prieta Earthquake.' (abstract) *Journal of Personality and Social Psychology,* 61(1): 115-121.

North, T. C., McCullagh, P. & Vu Tran, Z. 1990. 'Effect of Exercise on Depression.' *Exercise and Sports Sciences Reviews,* 80:379-416.

Otto, M. W., Reilly-Harrington, N. & Sachs, G. S. 2003. 'Psychoeducational and cognitive-behavioral strategies in the management of bipolar disorder.' (abstract) *Journal of Affective Disorders,* 73: 171-181.

Oubr, A. 2002. 'EEG Neurofeedback for Treating Psychiatric Disorder.' *Psychiatric Times,* XIX, no 2 (Feb 2002).

Paquette, A. 2016. *I Have Bipolar Disorder and I Take Medication.* http://www.bphope.com [accessed 12.08.17]

Parekh, R. *rev: APA* 2017. APA Bipolar Disorders webpage. http;//www.psychiatry.org/patients-families/bipolar-disorders/what-are-bipolar-disorders [accessed 20.04.18]

Parker, G., Gibson, N. A., Brothcie, H., Heruc, G., Rees, A-M. & Hadzi-Pavlovic, D. 2006. 'Omega-3 Fatty Acids and Mood Disorders.' *American Journal of Psychiatry,* 163:969-978.

Perlman, C. A., Johnson, S. L. & Mellman, T. A. 2006.'The Prospective Impact of Sleep Duration on Depression and Mania.' (abstract) *Bipolar Disorders,* 8:271-274.

Perry, A., Tarrier, N., Morris, R., McCarthy, E. & Limb, K. 1999. 'Randomized Controlled Trial of Efficacy of Teaching Patients with Bipolar Disorder to Identify Early Symptoms of Relapse and Obtain Treatment.' *British Medical Journal,* 318(7177): 149-153.

Perugi, G., Akiskal, H. S., Ramacciotti, S., Nassini, S., Toni, C., Milanfranchi, A. & Musetti, L. (abstract) 'Depressive comorbidity of panic, social phobic, and obsessive-compulsive disorders re-examined: is there a bipolar II connection?' (abstract) *Journal of Psychiatric Research,* 33:53-61.

Quest, P. 2016. *Reiki for Life.* Tarcher Perigee: New York, NY

Railton, D. 2016. *Natural Remedies for Treating Bipolar Disorder.* Medical News Today. http://www.medicalnewstoday.com/articles/314435.php [accessed 05.08.17].

Regier, D. A., Farmer, M. E., Rae, D. S., Locke, B. Z., Keith, S. J., Judd, L. L. & Goodwin, F. K. 1990. 'Comorbidity of Mental Disorders with Alcohol and Other Drug Abuse: Results from the Epidemiologic Catchment Area Study.' (abstract) *Journal of the American Medical Association,* 264:2511-2518.

Rethink Mental Illness. *Antidepressants-About.* https://www.rethink.org/diagnosis-treatment/medications/antidepressants/about [accessed 18.08.17]

Rethink Mental Illness. *Antipsychotics.* https://www.rethink.org/diagnosis-treatment/medications/antipsychotics [accessed [18.08.17]

Rethink Mental Illness. *Mood Stabilisers.* https://www.rethink.org/diagnosis-treatment/medications/mood-stabilisers [accessed 18.08.17]

Rogers, P. J., Appleton, K. M., Kessler, D., Peters, T. J., Gannell, D., Hayward, R. C., Heatherley, S. V., Christian, L. M., McNaughton, S. A. & Ness, A. R. 2008. 'No Effect of n-3 Long-Chain Polyunsaturated Fatty Acid (EPA and DHA) Supplementation on Depressed Mood and Cognitive Function: A Randomised Controlled Trial.' *British Journal of Nutrition,* 99:421-431.

Sachs, G. S., Thase, M. E., Otto, M. W., Bauer, M., Miklowitz, D., Wisniewski, S. R. *et al.* 2003. 'Rationale, Design, and Methods of the Systematic Treatment Enhancement Program for Bipolar Disorder (STEP-BD).' (abstract) *Biological Psychiatry,* 53(11):1028-1042.

Sapp, M. 1994. 'The Effects of Guided Imagery on Reducing the Worry and Emotionality Components of Test Anxiety.' (abstract) *Journal of Mental Imagery,* 18(3-4):165-179.

Sarris, J., Mischoulon, D. & Schweitzer, I. 2011. 'Adjunctive Nutraceuticals with Standard Pharmaceuticals in Bipolar Disorder: A Systematic Review of Clinical Trials.' (abstract) *Bipolar Disorders,* 13: 454-465.

Serretti, A., Mandelli, L., Lattuada, E., Cusin, C. & Smeraldi, E. 2002. 'Clinical and Demographic Features of Mood Disorder Subtypes.' (abstract) *Psychiatry Research,* 112(3): 195-210.

Shabbir, F., Patel, A., Mattison, C. Bose, S., Krishnamohan, R., Sweeney, E., Sandhu, S., Nel., W., Rais, A., Sandhu, R., Ngu, N. & Sharma, S. 2013. 'Effect of Diet on Serotonergic Transmission in Depression'. (abstract) *Neurochemistry International,* 62:324-329.

Simon, N. M., Otto, M. W., Wisniewski, S. R., Fossey, M., Sagduyu, K., Frank, E. Sachs, G. S., Nierenberg, A. A., Thase M. E. & Pollack, M. H. 2004. 'Anxiety Disorder Comorbidity in Bipolar Disorder Patients: Data from the First 500 Participants in the Systematic Treatment Enhancement Program for Bipolar Disorder (STEP-BD).' *American Journal of Psychiatry,* 161(12):2222-2229.

Srinivasan, V., Smits, M., Spence, W., Lowe, A. D., Kayumov, L., Pandi-Perumal, S. R., Parry, B. & Cardinali, D. P. 2006. 'Melatonin in Mood Disorders.' (abstract) *World Journal of Biological Psychiatry,* 7:138-151.

Stahl, L. A., Begg, D. P. Weisinger, R. S. & Sinclair, A. J. 2008. 'The Role of Omega-3 Fatty Acids in Mood Disorders.' (abstract) *Current Opion in Investigational Drugs,* 9:57-64.

Suppes, T. & Keck, P. E. 2005. *Bipolar Disorder: Treatment and Management.* Compact Clinicals: Kansas City.

Teasdale, J. D., Segal, V., Williams, J. M., Ridgeway, V. A., Soulsby, J. M. & Lau, M. A. 2000. 'Prevention of Relapse/Recurrence in Major Depression in Mindfulness-Based Cognitive Therapy,' *Journal of Consulting and Clinical Psychology,* 68(4): 615-623.

Thase, M. E & Sachs, G. S. 2000. 'Bipolar depression: pharmacotherapy and related therapeutic strategies.' (abstract) *Biological Psychiatry,* 48:558-572.

Todd, G. 2016. *How to Live with a Bipolar Mind: Principles Learned from Personal Experience.* Amazon Fulfilment.

Vojta, C., Kinosian, B., Glick, H., Altshuler, L. & Bauer, M. S. 2001. 'Self-reported quality of life across mood states in bipolar disorder.' (abstract) *Comprehensive Psychiatry,* 42:190-195.

Vollebergh, W. A., Iederma, J., Bijl, R. V., de Graf, R., Smit, F. & Ormel, J. 2001. 'The structure and stability of common mental disorders: the NEMSIS study.' *Archives of General Psychiatry,* 58:597-603.

Wegner, D. M., Schneider, D. J., Carter, S. & White, T. L. 1987. 'Paradoxical Effects of Thought Suppression.' (abstract) *Journal of Personality and Social Psychology,* 53(1):5-13.

Wehr, T. A. & Goodwin, F. K. 1979. 'Rapid cycling in manic depressives induced by tricyclic antidepressants.' (abstract) *Archives of General Psychiatry,* 36:555-559.

Wehr, T. A., Sack, D. A> & Rosenthal, N. E. 1987. 'Sleep Reduction as a Final Common Pathway in the Genesis of Mania.' (abstract) *American Journal of Psychiatry,* 114(2): 201-204.

Wildes, J. E. Marcus, M. D. & Fagiolini, A. 2006. 'Obesity in Patients with Bipolar Disorder: A Biopsychosocial-Behavioral Model'. *Journal of Clinical Psychiatry,* 67:904-915.

Wooldridge, D. 2016. *Fear is My Co-Pilot: A Memoir.* DP & PW Publishing: Mesa, AZ.

Wu, L.H. & Dunner, D. L. 1993. 'Suicide attempts in rapid cycling bipolar disorder patients.' (abstract) *Journal of Affective Disorders,* 29:57-61.

Yatham, L.N., Kennedy, S. H., O'Donovan, C., Parikh, S., MacQueen, G., McIntyre, R., Sharma, V., Silverstone, P., Alda, M., Baruch, P., Beaulieu, S., Daigneault, A., Milev, R., Young, L. T., Ravindran, A., Schaffer, A., Connolly, M. & Gorman, C. P. 2005. 'Canadian Network for Mood and Anxiety Treatments (CANMAT) guidelines for management of patients with bipolar disorder: consensus and controversies.' (abstract) *Bipolar Disorders,* 7(3):5-69.

Young, T.L., Cooke, R. G., Robb, J. C., Levitt, A. J. & Joffe, R. T. 1993. 'Anxious and non-anxious bipolar disorder.' (abstract) *Journal of Affective Disorders,* 29:49-52.

Zaretsky, A. E., Segal, Z. V. & Gemar, M. 1999. 'Cognitive Therapy for Bipolar Depression: A Pilot Study.' *Canadian Journal of Psychiatry,* 44(5): 491-494.

Useful websites

www.bipolarhappens.com

www.bipolarlab.com

www.bipolaruk.org

www.bphope.com

www.healthline.com/health/bipolar-disorder

www.medicalnewstoday.com

www.moodtracker.com

Printed in Great Britain
by Amazon